Plant-Based Cookbook for Athletes

A Simple and Effective Guide to Learn how to Fuel Your Workouts, Build Muscle, Improve Performance and Increase Vitality

75 High-Protein Vegan Recipes with Pictures and 28-Day Meal Plan

Michael Gill

*To all athletes and health enthusiasts
excited to embrace the Plant-Based Lifestyle*

For the Planet, for the animals, and for Yourself!

Table of Contents

Introduction

Athlete Getting Started On A Vegan Diet

Common misunderstandings among many people—even in the health and fitness industry is that anyone who switches to a vegan diet will automatically become super healthy. There are plenty of vegan junk foods out there, such as frozen veggie pizza and non-dairy ice cream, which can really kill your health goals if you eat them all the time. Engaging in healthy foods is the only way you can reap health benefits.

On the other side, certain vegan snacks play a role in keeping you focused. They should be consumed in moderation, sparingly and in small bits.

Decide What a Vegan Diet Means for You

The first step is to make a determination on how to organize your vegan diet to help you move from your present culinary viewpoint. This is really unique, something that ranges from individual to individual. While some people choose not to consume any animal products at all, others make do with tiny bits of dairy or food at times. It really is up to you to decide what and how you want your vegan diet to look like. Perhaps notably, you have to make a large portion of your diet from whole vegan foods.

Understand What You Are Eating

Okay, now that you've made the decision, your next move on your side part requires a lot of study. What do we mean by that? Okay, if this is your first time trying out the vegan diet, the amount of foods containing animal products, particularly packaged foods, will shock you. You will find yourself cultivating the custom of reading tags when shopping. It points out that many pre-packaged foods contain animal products, and you need to keep a close eye on the packaging of the ingredients if you just want to stick to plant products for your new diet. You may have decided to allow a certain number of animal products in your diet; well, you'll just have to look out for foods filled with fats, carbohydrates, salt, preservatives, and other things that may affect your healthy diet.

Find Revamped Versions of Your Favorite Recipes

I'm sure you have plenty of favorite dishes, not necessarily vegan. For most people, leaving everything behind is usually the most difficult part. Nonetheless, there is still a way to meet you halfway. Take some time to think about those things you want that are not based on plants. Think along the lines of taste, shape, consistency, and so on; and search for substitutes throughout the diet based on food plants that can do what you're lacking.

Build a Support Network

Building a new routine is complicated, but it doesn't have to be. Find some friends that are glad to be with you in this lifestyle, or even family members. This will help you stay focused and motivated by having a form of emotional support and openness. You can do fun things like try out and share new recipes with these mates or even hit up restaurants offering a variety of vegan options. You can even go one step further and look up local vegan social media groups to help you expand your knowledge and support network.

Getting to the root of a vegan diet

You can find so many fascinating things to learn and do, but for now I'm going to take you to the basics and ask you which foods to avoid.

Valuable vegetables

You'll find a whole variety of vegetables that you'll really get to know quite well when eating vegan.

If you're new to this, at the beginning, you're likely to stick to tried-and-true, popular veggies because they're going to feel healthy. These vegetables are a good start:

- Beets
- Carrots
- Kale

- Parsley, basil, and other herbs
- Spinach
- Squash

- Sweet potatoes
- Fantastic fruits

We all love it! You need to get on this train if you haven't because the fruits are delicious; sweet; full of sugar, color, and beautiful vitamins; and so, so good for you.

- Apples
- Mango
- Avocado
- Pineapple
- Bananas
- Raspberries
- Blueberries
- Strawberries
- Coconut
- Wonderful whole grains

Consuming whole grains of good quality is a healthy part of a diet based on vegetables. Don't worry; you can still have your pastas and breads, but the key word here is "whole." You don't want the real thing to be polished or stored. When purchasing these items, make sure that the only ingredient is the grain itself. While it is possible to purchase proper whole grains in packaging from the shelf, make sure that you double-check the label to confirm that it is indeed a whole grain (and just a whole grain).

Lovable legumes

It is important to learn to love legumes on a vegan diet as they are a fantastic source of food, protein, and energy. It may take you and your body to get used to them for a while, but they will soon be your friends— especially if you find out how fun it is to consume them in soups, salads, burgers, and other inventive foods. Some of the best things to start with here are:

- Black beans
- Lentils
- Chickpeas
- Split peas
- Kidney beans
- Notable nuts and seeds

A handful of nuts are good. But the thing with eating them on a vegan diet is to make sure they are raw and unsalted. Along with your other delicious vegan foods, you should feel free to eat them in moderation as long as you enjoy them in their natural state. Here's the best to start with:

- Almonds
- Cashews
- Chia seeds
- Flaxseeds

- Hempseeds
- Pumpkin seeds
- Sunflower seeds
- Walnuts

What is a Vegan?

The origins of vegetarianism date back to ancient times. But the term «Vegan» was first used in the 40s by Donald Watson, co-founder of the Vegan Society, to describe a lifestyle doctrine that man should live without exploiting animals.

The following decades saw substantial growth in the industrialization of food production and an increase in the nature of food. We seemed to move from a "garden to plate" life to a 'factory to plate". Food came out of convenient packets, which we threw away after eating the unhealthy contents, resulting in bad health for us and garbage and gasses for the planet.

By the 70s attitudes to health followed a trend toward a more natural lifestyle. Cultures blended many ideas from the East, and food production in western countries came under scrutiny. Along with a movement towards more compassionate living, people started to become critical of meat-eating and the way animals are treated when they are bred for food.

A move towards more natural food production methods for plants and animals started gaining awareness amongst the younger generations, who had to deal with the damage that unhealthy food production was causing to the earth, to plants and animals, and us.

Vegetarianism became a trend a growing trend in the west. But also, we now realize that some cultures have been traditionally vegetarian for thousands of years.

Veganism seems to have evolved from recognizing that even a vegetarian lifestyle still doesn't improve the risk of certain kinds of health issues and that even a vegetarian lifestyle doesn't eliminate the suffering caused to animals when they are used for what they produce. Vegetarianism has become a trend in the West. But also, we now realize that some cultures have been traditionally vegetarian for thousands of years.

The production of eggs still involves the battery farming of chickens. Cows are physically restrained for hours a day, not to mention the diet and medical intervention required to make them produce more milk than they are evolved to produce.

Veganism recognizes that any treatment of animals that raises them for the production of food and products involves some measure of suffering.

We will look at more specific aspects of veganism and a vegan dietary choice in this book.

Chapter 1:   The Protein Requirements

Protein Requirement and How to calculate protein RDA best for your body

Healthy protein is a vital nutrient; its intake is essential for the wellness of your muscle mass and, for the wellness of the heart. Consuming healthy protein can, also, aid you handle specific illness and sustain your weight-loss initiatives. The quantity of healthy protein you need to take in is based upon your weight, exercise, age and various other variables.

Computing the RDA for protein

To figure out just how much healthy protein you ought to be consuming, there is a simple formula: take your weight, which you most likely recognize in extra pounds, and then you need to transform it to kgs. The ordinary American male evaluates to have 195.7 extra pounds (matching approximately 88.77 kilos), while the typical American woman evaluates to have 168.5 extra pounds (which amounts to a concerning 75.21 kilos).

Considering that most individuals need to consume about 0.8 grams of healthy protein per kilo of body weight, this implies that the RDA formula is:

(0.8 grams of healthy protein) x (weight in kilos).

Provided this standard, many males should consider that they should have an intake of 71 grams of healthy protein daily, due to the fact that 0.8 x 88.77 = 71.016. Ladies should eat around 60 grams of healthy protein each day, considering that the equation gives 0.8 x 75.21 = 60.168.

You can additionally simply increase your weight in extra pounds by 0.36 grams of healthy protein if you are having problem computing your body weight in kilos. This would change the RDA formula to the following:

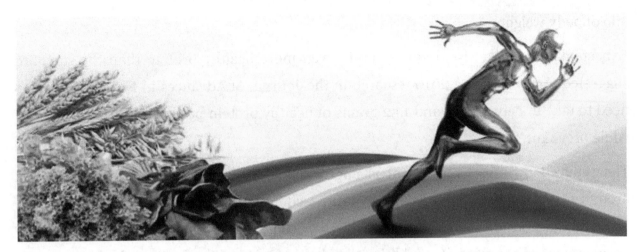

(0.36 grams of healthy protein) x (weight in extra pounds).

There is a selection of healthy protein consumption calculators offered online if you are not comfortable in computing your RDA for healthy protein by hand. You can use sites like the "United States Department of Agriculture's Dietary Reference Intakes Calculator".

Individuals who need more proteins

The RDA for healthy protein usually is 0.8 gram per kilo of body weight, lots of individuals can take in extra healthy protein safely. Professional athletes, for example, can eat as much of healthy protein as they desire as they burn a lot by exercising. Other individuals, like expecting females, nursing mothers and older generations additionally require eating even more of this nutrient.

The quantity of healthy protein you ought to eat as a professional athlete relies on the sort of exercise you take part in. Generally, individuals carrying out different workout routines ought to eat:

Minimum exercise (periodic stroll or extending): 1.0 gram of healthy protein per kilo of body weight.

Modest exercise (regular weight-lifting, quick strolling): 1.3 grams of healthy protein per kg of body weight.

Extreme training (professional athletes, routine joggers): 1.6 grams of healthy protein per kilo of body weight.

Expectant ladies, likewise, require eating even more healthy protein than the standard suggested. According to a 2016 research in the Journal of Advances in Nutrition, women need to take in between 1.2 and 1.52 grams of healthy protein per kilo of weight every day while pregnant.

The reduced quantity (1.2 grams) is appropriate for very early maternities stages of around 16 weeks, while the top quantity is advised for later maternities of about 36 weeks. The assumption of healthy protein by expectant ladies isn't just crucial for the development of the fetus; it is additionally vital in assisting the mother's body prepare to nurse their kids.

Vegetable Protein Diet: Do Vegetable Proteins Contain All The Essential Amino Acids?

Healthy proteins are the standard foundation of the body. They are comprised of amino acids and are required for the formation of muscular tissues, blood, skin, hair, nails, and the wellbeing of the interior body's organs. Besides water, healthy protein is one of the most abundant compounds in the body, and the majority of it is in the skeletal muscle mass.

Considering this, it is assuring to understand that according to the Dietary Guidelines for Americans between 2015-2020, most individuals obtain sufficient healthy protein daily. The very same record directs out that the consumption of fish and shellfish, and plant-based proteins such as seeds and nuts, are frequently lacking.

If you are an athlete, nonetheless, your healthy protein requirements might be somewhat greater considering that resistance training and endurance exercises can swiftly break down muscular tissue healthy protein.

If you are attempting to gain even more muscular tissue, you might assume that you require a lot more healthy protein, yet this isn't what you should do. There is proof that very strict professional athletes or exercisers might take in even more healthy protein (over 3 grams/kilograms daily), but for the typical exerciser, consumption of as much as 2 grams/per kg daily suffices for building muscle mass.

How Many Proteins Do You Really Need?

While the above standards offer you a general idea of where your healthy protein consumption needs to drop, determining the quantity of day-to-day healthy protein that's right for you, there is another method that can assist you in tweaking the previous results.

To identify your healthy protein requirements in grams (g), you need to initially determine your weight in kgs (kg) by separating your weight in pounds by 2.2.

Next off, choose the number of grams of healthy protein per kilo of bodyweight that is appropriate for you.

Use the reduced end of the array (0.8 g per kg) if you consider yourself to be healthy but not very active.

You should intake a more significant amount of protein (in between 1.2 and 2.0) if you are under tension, expecting, recuperating from a health problem, or if you are associated with extreme and constant weight or endurance training.

(You might require the recommendations of a physician or nutritional expert to assist you to establish this number).

Increase your weight in kg times the number of healthy protein grams per day.

For instance:

A 154-pound man that has as a routine exercising and lifting weights, but is not training at an elite degree:

154 lb/2.2 = 70 kg.

70 kg x 1.7 = 119 grams healthy protein each day.

Healthy protein as a percent of complete calories

An additional means to determine how much healthy protein you require is utilizing your everyday calorie consumption and the percentage of calories that will certainly originate from healthy protein.

Figure out exactly how many calories your body requires each day to keep your current weight.

Discover what your basic metabolic rate (BMR) is by utilizing a BMR calculator (often described as a basic power expense, or BEE, calculator).

Figure out the amount of calories you burn via day-to-day tasks and include that number to your BMR.

Next off, choose what portion of your diet plan will certainly originate from healthy protein. The percent you pick will certainly be based upon your objectives, physical fitness degree, age, type of body, and your metabolic rate. The Dietary Guidelines for Americans 2015-2020 advises that healthy protein represent something in between 10 percent and 35 percent for grownups suggested caloric intake.

Multiply that percentage by the complete variety of calories your body requires for the day to establish overall everyday calories from healthy protein.

Split that number by 4. (Quick Reference - 4 calories = 1 gram of healthy protein.)

For instance:

A 140-pound woman that eats 1800 calories each day consuming a diet plan having 20 percent of the total caloric intake consisting of healthy protein:

1800 x 0.20 = 360 calories from healthy protein.

360 calories/ 4 = 90 grams of healthy protein each day.

Compute daily protein need

To establish your day-to-day healthy protein requirement, increase your LBM by the suitable task degree.

- Less active (normally non-active): increase by 0.5.

- Light task (consists of strolling or horticulture): increase by 0.6.

- Modest (30 mins of a modest task, thrice weekly): increase by 0.7.

- Energetic (one hr of workout, 5 times regular): increase by 0.8.

- Really energetic (10 to 20 hrs of regular workout): increase by 0.9.

- Professional athlete (over 20 hrs of regular workout): increase by 1.0.

Based upon this approach, a 150-pound individual with an LBM of 105 would certainly need a day-to-day healthy protein amount that varies between 53 grams (if inactive) to 120 grams (if very active).

How To Calculate Your Protein Requirements?

It is crucial that we consume a sufficient amount of healthy protein each day to cover our body's requirements. Do you recognize just how much healthy protein you require?

Numerous professional athletes and other people that work out a lot assume that they ought to enhance their healthy protein consumption to assist them to shed their weight or construct even more muscle mass. It is real that the extra you work out, the higher your healthy protein requirement will undoubtedly be.

Healthy proteins are the standard foundation of the body. They are comprised of amino acids and are required for the formation of muscular tissues, blood, skin, hair, nails, and the wellbeing of the interior body's organs. Besides water, healthy protein is one of the most abundant compounds in the body, and the majority of it is in the skeletal muscle mass.

Considering this, it is assuring to understand that according to the Dietary Guidelines for Americans between 2015-2020, most individuals obtain sufficient healthy protein daily. The very same record directs out that the consumption of fish and shellfish, and plant-based proteins such as seeds and nuts, are frequently lacking.

If you are an athlete, nonetheless, your healthy protein requirements might be somewhat greater considering that resistance training and endurance exercises can swiftly break down muscular tissue healthy protein.

The basic standards for strength-trained and endurance professional athletes, according to the Academy of Nutrition and Dietetics, Dietitians of Canada, and the American College of Sports Medicine, is the recommended amount laying in between 1.2 and 2 grams of healthy protein per kg of body weight to achieve maximum efficiency and the health and wellness of the body.

If you are attempting to gain even more muscular tissue, you might assume that you require a lot healthier protein, yet this isn't what you should do. There is proof that very strict professional athletes or exercisers might take in even more healthy protein (over 3 grams/kilograms daily), but for the typical exerciser, consumption of as much as 2 grams/per kg daily suffices for building muscle mass.

When establishing your healthy protein requirements, you can either recognize a percent of overall day-to-day calories, or you can target in detail the number of grams of healthy protein to eat each day.

Percent of daily calories

Present USDA nutritional standards recommend that adult males and females should take an amount in between 10 and 35 percent of their overall calories intake from healthy protein. To obtain your number and to track your consumption, you'll require to understand the number of calories you eat daily.

To keep a healthy and balanced weight, you need to take in about the same variety of calories that you burn daily.

Just increase that number by 10 percent and by 35 percent to obtain your variety when you understand precisely how many calories you take in daily.

As an example, a male that eats 2,000 calories each day would more or less require to eat between 200 to 700 calories every day of healthy protein.

Healthy protein grams each day

As an option to the portion method, you can target the specific amount of healthy protein grams each day.

One straightforward method to obtain an amount of healthy protein grams daily is to equate the percent array into a particular healthy protein gram variety. The mathematical formula for this is very easy.

Each gram of healthy protein consists of 4 calories, so you will just need to split both calorie array numbers by 4.

A guy that consumes 2,000 calories daily must take in between 200 and 700 calories from healthy protein or 50 to 175 grams of healthy protein.

There are various other methods to obtain a much more specific number which might consider lean muscular tissue mass and/or exercise degree.

You can establish your fundamental healthy protein requirement as a percent of your complete day-to-day calorie consumption or as a series of healthy protein grams daily.

Healthy protein needs based on weight and activity

The ordinary adult demands a minimum of 0.8 grams of healthy protein per kg of body weight each day. One kg equates to 2.2 extra pounds, so an individual that has 165 extra pounds or 75 kg would more or less require around 60 grams of healthy protein daily.

Your healthy protein requirements might raise if you are very active. The Academy of Nutrition and Dietetics, American College of Sports Medicine and the Dietitians of Canada, recommend that professional athletes require even more healthy protein.

They recommend that endurance professional athletes (those that often take part in sports like running, biking, or swimming) take in 1.2 to 1.4 grams of healthy protein per kilo of body weight daily which equates to 0.5 to 0.6 grams of healthy protein per extra pound of body weight.

The companies recommend that strength-trained professional athletes (that engage in exercises like powerlifting or weightlifting often) take in 1.6 to 1.7 grams of healthy protein per kg of body weight. This equates to 0.7 to 0.8 grams of healthy protein per extra pound of body weight.

Healthy protein needs based on lean body mass

A new approach of finding out how much healthy protein you require is focused on the degree of the exercise (how much energy you spend) and your lean body mass. Some professionals really feel that this is an exact extra method because our lean body mass needs extra healthy protein for upkeep than fat.

Lean body mass (LBM) is merely the quantity of bodyweight that is not fat. There are various methods to identify your lean body mass, yet the most convenient is to deduct your body fat from your overall body mass.

You'll require to establish your body fat percent. There are various methods to obtain the number of your body fat consisting of screening with skin calipers, BIA ranges, or DEXA scans. You can approximate your body fat with the following calculating formula.

To determine your overall body fat in extra pounds, you will need to increase your body weight by the body fat portion. If you evaluate yourself to be 150 pounds and that your fat percent is 30, then 45 of those bodyweight pounds would certainly be fat (150 x 30% = 45).

Compute lean body mass. Merely deduct your body fat weight from your overall body weight. Utilizing the exact same instance, the lean body mass would certainly be 105 (150 - 45 = 105).

Chapter 2:   Why Choose A Vegan Diet

Why Go Vegan?

It's an ideal opportunity to stop the possibility that eating a veggie lover, vegetarian, or plant-based diet and being a solid, fit competitor are fundamentally unrelated.

A veggie lover or vegetarian diet for continuance competitors is truly not the same as a typical (sound) diet, with the exemption, obviously, of the meat and creature items. If you're changing from eating McDonald's consistently, then sure, it will take some becoming acclimated to. In any case, if you eat bunches of nutritious, whole foods all things considered, there truly aren't too numerous alterations you have to make to go veggie lover, and from that point, to go vegetarian or plant-based.

You can accept it to the extent you need, and some veggie lover and vegetarian competitors incline toward crude and sans gluten eats less carbs, referring to much more prominent energy gains.

Obviously, you don't need to take it that far to see the advantages. There are contrasting degrees of well-being in plant-based weight control plans, and mine incorporates a great deal of delectable cooked foods that individuals following progressively customary diets would eat.

The Plant-Based Diet for Muscle Gain and Strength

The equivalent can be said about going plant-based when you will probably include muscle, or basically get swollen.

In any case, when that is the objective, there are a couple of interesting points about your sustenance (precisely like there would be if you were attempting to include muscle a non-veggie lover diet):

    a. Macronutrient proportions that fit your particular body and objectives.

    b. Understanding your caloric needs.

Furthermore, having an appropriate exercise intend to go with your food technique.

Where Do You Get Your Protein?

Ok truly, every veggie lover competitor's preferred inquiry.

The appropriate response is that protein is in all plant foods, only for the most part in lower amounts. In any case, in case you're eating a balanced plant-based diet with a sound mix of beans, nuts, and seeds, you'll for the most part experience no difficulty getting all that anyone could need protein from whole plant foods.

From the start, it might require some cognizant exertion to ensure you get a sound measure of protein in each feast, however it isn't so difficult.

In case you're forcefully attempting to manufacture muscle, or in case you're simply worried about your protein levels, there's consistently the alternative for plant-based protein powders, however the vast majority won't require them.

The food we devour is made out of substance aggravates that are separated into two fundamental classifications: macrovitamins and microvitamins.

Macrovitamins are the mixes we devour in the biggest amounts, and they incorporate protein, starches, and fat. Microvitamins, then again, are supplements required in little amounts to arrange a scope of physiological capacities. They incorporate vitamins and minerals.

Capitalizing on Macrovitamins

The macrovitamin class is the trick just for protein, sugars, and fats. These supplements are the fundamental structure squares we require from our diet to enable us to flourish, feel fulfilled, have enough energy, and assemble muscle and in general well-being. In case you're feeling the loss of any of these significant classifications, it can set you up for desires, malfood, constant disease, and a general longing to "stock up" on what your body is absent.

In some cases individuals overcompensate by over-expending a specific macrovitamin when one is absent. For instance, devouring a high-protein diet when you're missing carbs can be perilous. Eating an excessive amount of protein isn't really better; the body needs a healthy proportion of each of the three macrovitamins to flourish and endure.

Considering Protein In The Plant-Based World

Protein is the significant structure hinder the body uses to deliver things like muscle, hair, and nails and help with development and recovery of tissue. Also, it's fundamental to practically all significant elements of the body. Without it, our bodies would absolutely separate.

There are two kinds of proteins: complete and deficient. To be viewed as complete, a protein must contain each of the 22 amino acids, including the 8 fundamental amino acids (amino acids that your body can't create and that you should get from your diet). I show some extraordinary plant-based total proteins in the "Inspecting plant proteins" segment.

It's significant that you eat total proteins; else, you may encounter edema; weakness; misery; poor resistance; muscle loss; hair that is dark, free, or dropping out; low vitamin A levels; waterfalls; and that's just the beginning.

Proteins that are low in some fundamental amino acids are viewed as deficient. Yet, fortunately if you eat an assortment of inadequate plant-protein foods together, they go about as a total protein — for instance, dark coloured rice and chick-peas or almond butter on toast. Far and away superior news is that these foods don't need to be eaten around the same time — the body has an amino-corrosive bank that aggregates over two or three days, after which it joins and amasses the single amino acids to make total proteins.

Understanding What A Solid Body REQUIRES

As the World Health Organization has inquired about this subject, it has found that we need less protein than we recently suspected. When all is said in done, a healthy body requires in any event three to four servings of plant-based protein daily. This works out to a scope of around 20 to 60 grams every day. You don't need to go excessively insane attempting to apportion everything; the sort and mix of protein you devour is definitely more significant than the amount.

Not all proteins are made equivalent! Great proteins are simpler for your body to separate and retain, while terrible proteins, for example, prepared, manufactured, or cooked animal proteins (in which the amino acids have been separated), are progressively hard for your body to assimilate. Fortunately when you eat a plant-based diet, the chances of your protein falling into the "great" class are a lot higher than when you eat a animal based diet.

Looking At Plant Proteins

Plant protein is loaded with benefits: It's generally antacid shaping contrasted with animal protein (which means it nourishes the blood), low in fat, liberated from development hormones, simple to process, and better for the earth. Also, in spite of normal misguided judgments, the plant world offers a lot of wellsprings of protein. Finished plant-based proteins are found in foods like quinoas, hemp, chlorella, and soybeans. Believe it or not, many plant-based proteins are quite finished, so as long as you eat an assortment of them, you get what your body requires.

Here are a few wellsprings of plant-based protein:

- Beans: Fresh or canned natural beans, green and yellow split peas, dark beans, chickpeas, lentils, naval force beans, white beans

- Butters: Almond, pumpkin, cashew, sunflower

- Greens: Chlorella, spirulina, blue green growth, kale, chard

- Nuts: Almonds, cashews, pecans, walnuts, Brazil nuts, macadamia nuts

- Protein powders: Hemp, pea, dark coloured rice

- Seeds: Tahini, sunflower, pumpkin, sesame, flax, chia, quinoa, amaranth

- Soy: Sprouted tofu, tempeh, edamame

- Sprouts: Mung bean, adzuki, pea, sunflower, lentil

Some especially protein-stuffed plant foods incorporate spinach, which is 51 percent protein; mushrooms, tipping the scales at 35 percent; beans, which are 26 percent protein; and oats, which is at 16 percent.

Considering Carboriffic Plants

Starches are long chains of carbon that give energy in a period discharge style to guarantee a relentless glucose level. In opposition to what numerous individuals accept, high-sugar foods are not naturally stuffing. We believe that since they're comprised of sugars, and refined sugars, (for example, fructose) in overabundance can make you put on weight. As a general rule, sugars have not exactly a large portion of the calories found in fat. Furthermore, sugars have high convergences of protein and basic vitamins and minerals, including B vitamins, vitamin E, folate, calcium, selenium, iron, magnesium, and zinc. So yahoo — expedite the bread.

Research shows that ladies who eat starches recoup all the more rapidly from side effects of PMS. Carbs can go about as natural sedatives and are gainful for individuals with regular versatile issue and sadness.

The principle capacity of sugars is to give a wellspring of energy to your body. Every gram of starch gives around four kilocalories of energy. You need a steady stock of starches as glucose for every metabolic response to happen appropriately. Complex carbs additionally help the amino acids in protein to be consumed and utilized appropriately.

If you don't devour enough carbs, your body can go to fat or protein for energy. This isn't perfect because the transformation of fat to glucose can go just so rapidly and can cause a development of corrosive in the blood, making a condition known as ketosis.

Looking At Basic And Complex Carbs

It's critical to comprehend the various types of carbs and how to recognize them. The straightforward ones are the ones we need to limit so we can concentrate on the complex.

Straightforward Carbs

There are two sorts of basic starches: monosaccharides and disaccharides. Monosaccharides comprise of just one sugar, and models incorporate fructose, galactose, and glucose. Disaccharides comprise of two synthetically connected monosaccharides, and they come as lactose, maltose, and sucrose.

Foods that contain straightforward starches incorporate table sugar, items made with white flour, dairy items, whole natural product, fruit juice, jam, pop, and pack-matured oats. So it's quite clear that basic sugars ought to be jettisoned (with the exception of the whole fruit, obviously, as it contains fibre and numerous other superb supplements).

Complex Carbs

Complex starches have a higher healthy benefit than straightforward starches since they comprise of at least three sugars that are generally plentiful in fibre, vitamins, and minerals. As a result of their unpredictability, they take somewhat longer to process, and they don't raise glucose levels as fast as basic sugars. Complex starches go about as the body's fuel and they con-tribute fundamentally to energy creation. They're significant in the retention of specific minerals and the development of unsaturated fats.

Foods that contain complex starches incorporate oats, dark coloured rice, sweet potatoes, and vegetables.

Getting ENOUGH Of The Privilege Carbs

Antiquated grains are probably the most seasoned foods on earth. They've been utilized for a huge number of years and are a superb wellspring of complex sugars, which help control hunger. These grains likewise contain phytochemicals, which can help lower cholesterol and forestall malignant growth and different infections. When joined with vegetables and vegetables, whole grains give total sustenance!

Here are some helpful grains how-to:

- Consume one to two servings every day (½ cup or one cut of bread is identical to one segment of grain).

- Focus on sans gluten whole grains (dark coloured rice, quinoa, millet, amaranth, and buckwheat). These sorts of grain are a lot simpler to process and contain an assortment of supplements. They additionally cook rapidly.

- Choose options in contrast to wheat (spelt, kamut, oats, grain, and rye).

- Choose grew grain items.

- Use these grains in their whole structure or as ground flours, in pastas, breads, wraps, and saltines.

- Presently, grains aren't the main game around. Other helpful wellsprings of complex starches include:

- Fruits: Organic, regular, low-glycemic natural products, for example, apples, berries, and pears

- Legumes: Lentils, chickpeas, split peas, kidney beans, pinto beans, and dark beans

- Starchy vegetables: Squash, sweet potatoes, yams, carrots, and beets

Planning Suppers With Complex Sugars

Carbs are a major supplement classification and will in general be the place numerous individuals get the greater part of their calories. Since sugars make up such a solid and enormous piece of a plant-based way of life, I've recorded some brisk thoughts here for supper planning

Breakfast

- Porridge: Scottish or steel-cut oats absorbed water medium-term and cooked in the first part of the day on delicate warmth for 5 to 10 minutes; include rice milk and some maple syrup and cinnamon (and splashed dried fruits)

- Fresh, regular fruit with natively constructed granola and coconut yogurt or then again cashew cream

- Whole-grain grew bread or rice saltines with nut butter

- Whole-grain hotcakes with crisp foods grown from the ground cream

Lunch Or Supper

- Spelt or rye bread or wrap with hummus, beans, crude or barbecued veggies, avocado, and tempeh or tofu

- Brown rice with lentils or beans and steamed veggies

- Grain servings of mixed greens and pilafs (quinoa, wild rice, grain) with vinaigrette

- Baked yam or winter squash with green verdant serving of mixed greens, steamed veggies, and beans or tempeh

Minimal-Craving Suppers

- Saturated oats or porridge with nectar or coconut nectar

- Plain brown rice with olive oil and steamed veggies

- Quinoa with olive oil, flax oil, or tahini

Avoiding the awful carbs

Notwithstanding ensuring you expend complex starches as a major aspect of your reasonable plant-based diet, you ought to stay away from the two downright awful carbs totally: refined sugars and flours and counterfeit sugars. They not just straightforwardly sway your glucose levels by activating sharp spikes and drops but at the same time are "unfilled" as far as supplements and amazingly irresistible.

Refined sugar and flour are the most processed type of carbs you can expend, and shockingly they're all over the place. Refined sugars stow away on display, so you need to truly be on your game! Notwithstanding avoiding the conspicuous white granulated and powdered sugars, avoid ingredients like:

- High-fructose corn syrup

- Wheat flour

- Enriched flour

- Sugar

Fake sugars are synthetically made-up sugars that can neutralize you. They can fool your body into believing you're getting some type of sugar, yet rather they cause you to hunger for more starches. Also, they're amazingly risky to your blood, liver, and sensory system. These incorporate sucralose and aspartame, which are basic in diet beverages and foods.

Eating Greasy Plants

Fat gets negative criticism. We consider it the adversary, isn't that right? We attempt to keep away from it no matter what. We trust it's the wellspring of all abhorrent (and expanding waistlines), yet here's a newsflash: We need fat. Fats are our companions. Or possibly some of them — with some restraint — are. Let's separate companion from enemy.

The ones YOU SHOULD know: SATURATED, mono, poly

Saturated, monounsaturated, and polyunsaturated fats are the three most regular types of fat that you experience in the plant world. Fats are ordered by their thickness and the quantity of carbons in a chain. Without getting excessively confused, the more carbons a fat has, the more saturated it is. Here's a little breakdown, beginning with the most saturated of fats:

Saturated fats:

- Don't ordinarily go malodorous, in any event, when warmed for cooking

- Are made in our bodies from sugars

- Constitute at any rate 50 percent of our cell layers, giving cells firmness and honesty

- Are required for calcium to be successfully consolidated into the skeletal framework

- Protect the liver from liquor and different poisons

- Enhance insusceptible capacity

- Are required for the best possible utilization of fundamental unsaturated fats (EFAs)

- Plant-based sources: coconut oil and palm oil

Monounsaturated fats:

- Tend to be fluid at room temperature
- Don't go rank effectively and can be utilized in cooking at moderate temperatures
- Plant-based sources: olive oil, almonds, walnuts, cashews, peanuts, avocados

Polyunsaturated fats:

- Contain omega-3 and omega-6 unsaturated fats
- Are fluid in any event, when refrigerated
- Should never be warmed
- Plant-based sources: pecans, chia, hemp, and flax

Most "politically right" sustenance (which means what the administration needs you to eat) depends on the supposition that we ought to decrease and in a perfect world kill our intake of fats — especially saturated fats — from animal sources since they're to be faulted for things like coronary illness. In any case, don't let your plant-based diet hush you into an incorrect conviction that all is well with the world. To an ever increasing extent, we're finding that it's less the saturated fats that are to be faulted yet rather the processed food of the present current industry and those trans fats covered up in many items. That implies even though you're eating plant-based, you despite everything are in risk for coronary illness and other well-being complexities if you devour a lot of butter, shortening, refined oils and sugars, and prepared foods when all is said in done.

Fundamental fats VERSUS fats to avoid

We have to devour various fats consistently from a wide assortment of sources. The food they give is fundamental to your body and your well-being.

Chapter 3: 7 Benefits of A Vegan Diet

Benefits Of Veganism In The Field Of Sport

I think it is finally clear how it is possible to get the right amount of protein on a vegan diet, even for all those who play competitive sports. The most interesting thing is that anyone who inquire properly will also find very interesting all the benefits of a plant-based lifestyle.

But what are the advantages that an athlete can get through a vegan diet?

1. Improvement of muscle metabolism

2. Greater strength

3. Reduced muscle pain

4. Less fatigue

5. Best recovery time

6. Decrease in the rate of inflammation

7. More energy

Those who switch to a vegan diet get immediate benefits on their strength and note a better and faster muscle development. For an athlete also should not be underestimated the advantage of boosting the immune system, since it allows him to get sick less frequently and therefore, he can focus better on training.

Furthermore, in vegan nutrition there are no foods that are in fact pro-inflammatory, such as meat and dairy products, rich in cholesterol and saturated fats.

However, we should not make the mistake of believing that it suffices to be vegan so that everything goes well. Like any kind of nutrition, we need to make sure to incorporate a good variety of nutrient-rich food sources.

It is a good idea to structure a good personalized plan of weekly meals in order to be sure of assimilating everything the body needs. It is also good to feed several times a day and tossing away the famous rule of "three meals a day." High-end athletes eat up to 8-9 times a day, following their personalized nutritional program.

This is the only way we can be sure to provide the body with a varied balance of carbohydrates, proteins and fats, as well as fresh fruit and vegetables.

Since a nutrition program is always personal and therefore suitable only for a single individual, in this book I will not give you such a nutritional plan precisely because it may not be suitable for your individual person. I don't know you and I don't know if you are a beginner or an accomplished athlete, I don't know if you weigh 80 kg or 120 kg, I don't know your height or the sport you play. But I will make sure that you don't lose the pleasure for eating, providing you with tasty and nutritious recipes so you can enjoy the food as much as you enjoy your training. Food and workout go hand in hand, the more these activities are performed well and with pleasure, the better the results will be.

Before moving on to the recipes, let us briefly examine the protein content of some plant food.

Chapter 4:   Breakfast Recipes

1. Chocolate PB Smoothie

Preparation time: 5 minutes

Cooking time: 0 minutes

Servings: 4

Ingredients

1 banana

¼ cup rolled oats, or 1 scoop plant protein powder

1 tablespoon flaxseed, or chia seeds

1 tablespoon unsweetened cocoa powder

1 tablespoon peanut butter, or almond or sunflower seed butter

1 tablespoon maple syrup (optional)

1 cup alfalfa sprouts, or spinach, chopped (optional)

½ cup non-dairy milk (optional)

1 cup water

Optional

1 teaspoon maca powder

1 teaspoon cocoa nibs

Directions

Purée everything in a blender until smooth, adding more water (or non-dairy milk) if needed. Add bonus boosters, as desired. Purée until blended.

Nutrition: calories: 474; protein: 13g; total fat: 16g; carbohydrates: 79g; fiber: 18g

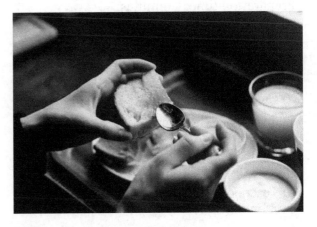

2. Orange French Toast

Preparation time: 15 minutes

Cooking time: 10 minutes

Servings: 4

Ingredients

3 very ripe bananas

1 cup unsweetened nondairy milk

Zest and juice of 1 orange

1 teaspoon ground cinnamon

¼ Teaspoon grated nutmeg

4 slices french bread

1 tablespoon coconut oil

Directions

In a blender, combine the bananas, almond milk, orange juice and zest, cinnamon, and nutmeg and blend until smooth. Pour the mixture into a 9-by-13-inch baking dish. Soak the bread in the mixture for 5 minutes on each side.

While the bread soaks, heat a griddle or sauté pan over medium-high heat. Melt the coconut oil in the pan and swirl to coat. Cook the bread slices until golden brown on both sides, about 5 minutes each. Serve immediately.

3. Oatmeal Raisin Breakfast Cookie

Preparation time: 5 minutes

Cooking time: 15 minutes

Servings: 2 cookies

Ingredients

½ Cup rolled oats

1 tablespoon whole-grain flour

½ Teaspoon baking powder

1 to 2 tablespoons brown sugar

½ Teaspoon pumpkin pie spice or ground cinnamon (optional)

¼ Cup unsweetened applesauce, plus more as needed

2 tablespoons raisins, dried cranberries, or vegan chocolate chips

Directions

In a medium bowl, stir together the oats, flour, baking powder, sugar, and pumpkin pie spice (if using). Stir in the applesauce until thoroughly combined. Add another 1 to 2 tablespoons of applesauce if the mixture looks too dry (this will depend on the type of oats used).

Shape the mixture into 2 cookies. Put them on a microwave-safe plate and heat on high power for 90 seconds. Alternatively, bake on a small tray in a 350°f oven or toaster oven for 15 minutes. Let cool slightly before eating.

Nutrition (2 cookies): calories: 175; protein: 74g; total fat: 2g; saturated fat:0g; carbohydrates: 39g; fiber: 4g

4. Berry Beetsicle Smoothie

Preparation time: 3 minutes

Cooking time: 0minutes

Servings: 1

Ingredients

½ Cup peeled and diced beets

½ Cup frozen raspberries

1 frozen banana

1 tablespoon maple syrup

1 cup unsweetened soy or almond milk

Directions

Combine all the Ingredients in a blender and blend until smooth.

5. Blueberry Oat Muffins

Preparation time: 10 minutes

Cooking time: 20 minutes

Servings: 12 mufins

Ingredients

2 tablespoons coconut oil or vegan margarine, melted, plus more for preparing the muffin tin

1 cup quick-cooking oats or instant oats

1 cup boiling water

½ Cup nondairy milk

¼ Cup ground flaxseed

1 teaspoon vanilla extract

1 teaspoon apple cider vinegar

1½ cups whole-grain flour

½ Cup brown sugar

2 teaspoons baking soda

Pinch salt

1 cup blueberries

Directions

Preheat the oven to 400°f.

Coat a muffin tin with coconut oil, line with paper muffin cups, or use a nonstick tin.

In a large bowl, combine the oats and boiling water. Stir so the oats soften. Add the coconut oil, milk, flaxseed, vanilla, and vinegar and stir to combine. Add the flour, sugar, baking soda, and salt. Stir until just combined. Gently fold in the blueberries. Scoop the muffin mixture into the prepared tin, about ⅓ cup for each muffin.

Bake for 20 to 25 minutes, until slightly browned on top and springy to the touch. Let cool for about 10 minutes. Run a dinner knife around the inside of each cup to loosen, then tilt the muffins on their sides in the muffin wells so air gets underneath. These keep in an airtight container in the refrigerator for up to 1 week or in the freezer indefinitely.

Nutrition (1muffin): calories: 174; protein: 5g; total fat: 3g; saturated fat:2g; carbohydrates: 33g; fiber: 4g

6. Quinoa Applesauce Muffins

Preparation time: 10 minutes

Cooking time: 15 minutes

Servings: 5

Ingredients

2 tablespoons coconut oil or margarine, melted, plus more for coating the muffin tin

¼ Cup ground flaxseed

½ Cup water

2 cups unsweetened applesauce

½ Cup brown sugar

1 teaspoon apple cider vinegar

2½ cups whole-grain flour

1½ cups cooked quinoa

2 teaspoons baking soda

Pinch salt

½ Cup dried cranberries or raisins

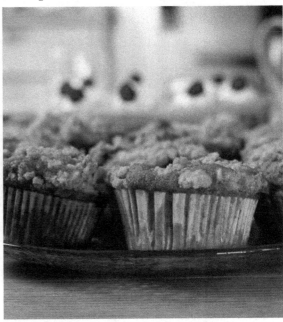

Directions

Preheat the oven to 400°f.

Coat a muffin tin with coconut oil, line with paper muffin cups, or use a nonstick tin. In a large bowl, stir together the flaxseed and water. Add the applesauce, sugar, coconut oil, and vinegar. Stir to combine. Add the flour, quinoa, baking soda, and salt, stirring until just combined. Gently fold in the cranberries without stirring too much. Scoop the muffin mixture into the prepared tin, about ⅓ cup for each muffin.

Bake for 15 to 20 minutes, until slightly browned on top and springy to the touch. Let cool for about 10 minutes. Run a dinner knife around the inside of each cup to loosen, then tilt the muffins on their sides in the muffin wells so air gets underneath. These keep in an airtight container in the refrigerator for up to 1 week or in the freezer indefinitely.

Per serving(1muffin): calories: 387; protein: 7g; total fat: 5g; saturated fat: 2g; carbohydrates: 57g; fiber: 8g

7. Pumpkin Pancakes

Preparation time: 15 minutes

Cooking time: 15 minutes

Servings: 4

Ingredients

2 cups unsweetened almond milk

1 teaspoon apple cider vinegar

2½ cups whole-wheat flour

2 tablespoons baking powder

½ Teaspoon baking soda

1 teaspoon sea salt

1 teaspoon pumpkin pie spice or ½ teaspoon ground -cinnamon plus ¼ teaspoon grated -nutmeg plus ¼ teaspoon ground allspice

½ Cup canned pumpkin purée

1 cup water

1 tablespoon coconut oil

Directions

In a small bowl, combine the almond milk and apple cider vinegar. Set aside.

In a bowl, whisk together the flour, baking powder, baking soda, salt, and pumpkin pie spice. In bowl, combine the almond milk mixture, pumpkin purée, and water, whisking to mix well. Mix the wet Ingredients to the dry Ingredients and fold together until the dry -Ingredients are just moistened.

In a nonstick pan or griddle over medium-high heat, melt the coconut oil and swirl to coat. Pour the batter into the pan ¼ cup at a time and cook until the pancakes are browned, about 5 minutes per side. Serve immediately.

8. Green Breakfast Smoothie

Preparation time: 10 minutes

Cooking time: 0 minutes

Servings: 2

Ingredients

½ Banana, sliced

2 cups spinach or other greens, such as kale

1 cup sliced berries of your choosing, fresh or frozen

1 orange, peeled and cut into segments

1 cup unsweetened nondairy milk

1 cup ice

Directions

In a blender, combine all the Ingredients.

Starting with the blender on low speed, begin blending the smoothie, gradually increasing blender speed until smooth. Serve immediately.

9. Blueberry And Chia Smoothie

Preparation time: 10 minutes

Cooking time: 0 minutes

Servings: 2

Ingredients

2 tablespoons chia seeds

2 cups unsweetened nondairy milk

2 cups blueberries, fresh or frozen

2 tablespoons pure maple syrup or agave

2 tablespoons cocoa powder

Directions:

Soak the chia seeds in the almond milk for 5 minutes.

In a blender, combine the soaked chia seeds, almond milk, blueberries, maple syrup, and cocoa powder and blend until smooth. Serve immediately.

10. Warm Maple and Cinnamon Quinoa

Preparation time: 5 minutes

Cooking time: 15 minutes

Servings: 4

Ingredients

1 cup unsweetened nondairy milk

1 cup water

1 cup quinoa, rinsed

1 teaspoon cinnamon

¼ Cup chopped pecans or other nuts or seeds, such as chia, sunflower seeds, or almonds

2 tablespoons pure maple syrup or agave

Directions:

In a medium saucepan over medium-high heat, bring the almond milk, water, and quinoa to a boil. Lower the heat to medium-low and cover. Simmer until the liquid is mostly absorbed and the quinoa softens, about 15 minutes.

Turn off the heat and allow to sit, covered, for 5 minutes. Stir in the cinnamon, pecans, and syrup. Serve hot.

11. Warm Quinoa Breakfast Bowl

Preparation time: 5 minutes

Cooking time: 0 minutes

Servings: 4

Ingredients

3 cups freshly cooked quinoa

1⅓ cups unsweetened soy or almond milk

2 bananas, sliced

1 cup raspberries

1 cup blueberries

½ Cup chopped raw walnuts

¼ Cup maple syrup

Directions:

Divide the Ingredients among 4 bowls, starting with a base of ¾ cup quinoa, ⅓ cup milk, ½ banana, ¼ cup raspberries, ¼ cup blueberries, and 2 tablespoons walnuts.

Drizzle 1 tablespoon of maple syrup over the top of each bowl.

12. Banana Bread Rice Pudding

Preparation time: 5 minutes

Cooking time: 50 minutes

Servings: 4

Ingredients

1cup brown rice

1½ cups water

1½ cups nondairy milk

3 tablespoons sugar (omit if using a sweetened nondairy milk)

2 teaspoons pumpkin pie spice or ground cinnamon

2 bananas

3 tablespoons chopped walnuts or sunflower seeds (optional)

Directions

In a medium pot, combine the rice, water, milk, sugar, and pumpkin pie spice. Bring to a boil over high heat, turn the heat to low, and cover the pot. Simmer, stirring occasionally, until the rice is soft and the liquid is absorbed. White rice takes about 20 minutes; brown rice takes about 50 minutes.

Smash the bananas and stir them into the cooked rice. Serve topped with walnuts (if using). Leftovers will keep refrigerated in an airtight container for up to 5 days.

Nutrition: calories: 479; protein: 9g; total fat: 13g; saturated fat: 1g; carbohydrates: 86g; fiber: 7g

13.Apple and Cinnamon Oatmeal

Preparation time: 10 minutes

Cooking time:10 minutes

Servings: 2

Ingredients

1¼ cups apple cider

1 apple, peeled, cored, and chopped

⅔ Cup rolled oats

1 teaspoon ground cinnamon

1 tablespoon pure maple syrup or agave
(optional)

Directions

In a medium saucepan, bring the apple cider
to a boil over medium-high heat. Stir in the
apple, oats, and cinnamon.

Bring the cereal to a boil and turn down heat
to low. Simmer until the oatmeal thickens, 3
to 4 minutes. Spoon into two bowls and
sweeten with maple syrup, if using. Serve
hot.

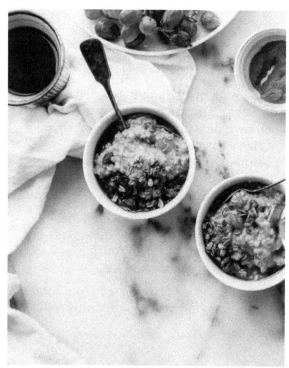

14.Mango Key Lime Pie Smoothie

Preparation time: 5 minutes

Cooking time: 0 minutes

Servings: 1

Ingredients

¼ Avocado

1 cup baby spinach

½ Cup frozen mango chunks

1 cup unsweetened soy or almond milk

Juice of 1 lime (preferably a key lime).

1 tablespoon maple syrup

Directions

Combine all the Ingredients in a blender and
blend until smooth. Enjoy immediately.

15.Spiced Orange Breakfast Couscous

Preparation time: 10 minutes

Cooking time: 10 minutes

Servings: 4

Ingredients

3 cups orange juice

1½ cups couscous

1 teaspoon ground cinnamon

¼ Teaspoon ground cloves

½ Cup dried fruit, such as raisins or apricots

½ Cup chopped almonds or other nuts or
seeds

Directions

In a small saucepan, bring the orange juice to
a boil. Add the couscous, cinnamon, and
cloves and remove from heat. Cover the pan
with a lid and allow to sit until the -couscous
softens, about 5 minutes.

Fluff the couscous with a fork and stir in the
dried fruit and nuts. Serve -immediately.

16. Breakfast Parfaits

Preparation time: 15 minutes

Cooking time: 0 minutes

Servings: 2

Ingredients

One 14-ounce can coconut milk, refrigerated overnight

1 cup granola

½ Cup walnuts

1 cup sliced strawberries or other seasonal berries

Directions

Pour off the canned coconut-milk liquid and retain the solids.

In two parfait glasses, layer the coconut-milk solids, granola, walnuts, and -strawberries. Serve immediately.

17. Sweet Potato And Kale Hash

Preparation time: 10 minutes

Cooking time: 15 minutes

Servings: 2

Ingredients

1 sweet potato

2 tablespoons olive oil

½ Onion, chopped

1 carrot, peeled and chopped

2 garlic cloves, minced

½ Teaspoon dried thyme

1 cup chopped kale

Sea salt

Freshly ground black pepper

Directions

Prick the sweet potato with a fork and microwave on high until soft, about 5 minutes. Remove from the microwave and cut into ¼-inch cubes.

In a large nonstick sauté pan, heat the olive oil over medium-high heat. Add the onion and carrot and cook until softened, about 5 minutes. Add the garlic and thyme and cook until the garlic is fragrant, about 30 seconds.

Add the sweet potatoes and cook until the potatoes begin to brown, about 7 -minutes. Add the kale and cook just until it wilts, 1 to 2 minutes. Season with salt and pepper. Serve immediately.

18. Delicious Oat Meal

Preparation time: 10 minutes

Cooking time: 6 hours

Servings: 4

Ingredients:

3 cups water

3 cups almond milk

1 and ½ cups steel oats

4 dates, pitted and chopped

1 teaspoon cinnamon, ground

2 tablespoons coconut sugar

½ Teaspoon ginger powder

A pinch of nutmeg, ground

A pinch of cloves, ground

1 teaspoon vanilla extract

Directions:

Put water and milk in your slow cooker and stir.

Add oats, dates, cinnamon, sugar, ginger, nutmeg, cloves and vanilla extract, stir, cover and cook on low for 6 hours.

Divide into bowls and serve for breakfast.

Enjoy!

Nutrition: calories 120, fat 1, fiber 2, carbs 3, protein 5

19. Breakfast Cherry Delight

Preparation time: 10 minutes

Cooking time: 8 hours and 10 minutes

Servings: 4

Ingredients:

2 cups almond milk

2 cups water

1 cup steel cut oats

2 tablespoons cocoa powder

1/3 cup cherries, pitted

¼ Cup maple syrup

½ Teaspoon almond extract

For the sauce:

2 tablespoons water

1 and ½ cups cherries, pitted and chopped

¼ Teaspoon almond extract

Directions:

Put the almond milk in your slow cooker.

Add 2 cups water, oats, cocoa powder, 1/3 cup cherries, maples syrup and ½ teaspoon almond extract.

Stir, cover and cook on low for 8 hours.

In a small pan, mix 2 tablespoons water with 1 and ½ cups cherries and ¼ teaspoon almond extract, stir well, bring to a simmer over medium heat and cook for 10 minutes until it thickens.

Divide oatmeal into breakfast bowls, top with the cherries sauce and serve.

Enjoy!

Nutrition: calories 150, fat 1, fiber 2, carbs 6, protein 5

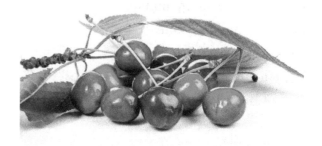

20. Crazy Maple and Pear Breakfast

Preparation time: 10 minutes

Cooking time: 9 hours

Servings: 2

Ingredients:

1 pear, cored and chopped

½ Teaspoon maple extract

2 cups coconut milk

½ Cup steel cut oats

½ Teaspoon vanilla extract

1 tablespoon stevia

¼ Cup walnuts, chopped for serving

Cooking spray

Directions:

Spray your slow cooker with some cooking spray and add coconut milk.

Also, add maple extract, oats, pear, stevia and vanilla extract, stir, cover and cook on low for 9 hours.

Stir your oatmeal again, divide it into breakfast bowls and serve with chopped walnuts on top.

Enjoy!

Nutrition: calories 150, fat 3, fiber 2, carbs 6, protein 6

21. Hearty French Toast Bowls

Preparation time: 10 minutes

Cooking time: 5 hours

Servings: 4

Ingredients:

1 and ½ cups almond milk

1 cup coconut cream

1 tablespoon vanilla extract

½ Tablespoon cinnamon powder

2 tablespoons maple syrup

¼ Cup spenda

2 apples, cored and cubed

½ Cup cranberries, dried

1 pound vegan bread, cubed

Cooking spray

Directions:

Spray your slow cooker with some cooking spray and add the bread.

Also, add cranberries and apples and stir gently.

Add milk, coconut cream, maple syrup, vanilla extract, cinnamon powder and splenda.

Stir, cover and cook on low for 5 hours.

Divide into bowls and serve right away.

Enjoy!

Nutrition: calories 140, fat 2, fiber 3, carbs 6, protein 2

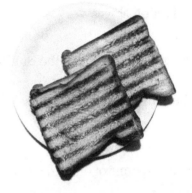

Chapter 5:   Lunch Recipes

22.   Cauliflower Latke

Preparation Time: 15 minutes

Cooking Time: 30 minutes

Servings: 4

Ingredients:

12 oz. cauliflower rice, cooked

1 egg, beaten

1/3 cup cornstarch

Salt and pepper to taste

¼ cup vegetable oil, divided

Chopped onion chives

Direction

Squeeze excess water from the cauliflower rice using paper towels.

Place the cauliflower rice in a bowl.

Stir in the egg and cornstarch.

Season with salt and pepper.

Pour 2 tablespoons of oil into a pan over medium heat.

Add 2 to 3 tablespoons of the cauliflower mixture into the pan.

Cook for 3 minutes per side or until golden.

Repeat until you've used up the rest of the batter.

Garnish with chopped chives.

Nutrition: Calories: 209 Total fat: 15.2g Saturated fat: 1.4g Cholesterol: 47mg Sodium: 331mg Potassium: 21mg Carbohydrates: 13.4g Fiber: 1.9g Sugar: 2g Protein: 3.4g

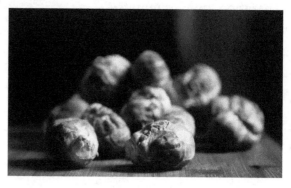

23.   Roasted Brussels Sprouts

Preparation Time: 30 minutes

Cooking Time: 20 minutes

Servings: 4

Ingredients:

1 lb. Brussels sprouts, sliced in half

1 shallot, chopped

1 tablespoon olive oil

Salt and pepper to taste

2 teaspoons balsamic vinegar

¼ cup pomegranate seeds

¼ cup goat cheese, crumbled

Direction:

Preheat your oven to 400 degrees F.

Coat the Brussels sprouts with oil.

Sprinkle with salt and pepper.

Transfer to a baking pan.

Roast in the oven for 20 minutes.

Drizzle with the vinegar.

Sprinkle with the seeds and cheese before serving.

Nutrition: Calories: 117 Total fat: 5.7g Saturated fat: 1.8g Cholesterol: 4mg Sodium: 216mg Potassium: 491mg Carbohydrates: 13.6g Fiber: 4.8g Sugar: 5g Protein: 5.8g

24. Brussels Sprouts & Cranberries Salad

Preparation Time: 10 minutes

Cooking Time: 0 minute

Servings: 6

Ingredients:

3 tablespoons lemon juice

¼ cup olive oil

Salt and pepper to taste

1 lb. Brussels sprouts, sliced thinly

¼ cup dried cranberries, chopped

½ cup pecans, toasted and chopped

½ cup vegan parmesan cheese, shaved

Direction

Mix the lemon juice, olive oil, salt and pepper in a bowl.

Toss the Brussels sprouts, cranberries and pecans in this mixture.

Sprinkle the Parmesan cheese on top.

Nutrition: Calories 245 Total Fat 18.9 g Saturated Fat 9 g Cholesterol 3 mg Sodium 350 mg Total Carbohydrate 15.9 g Dietary Fiber 5 g Protein 6.4 g Total Sugars 10 g Potassium 20 mg

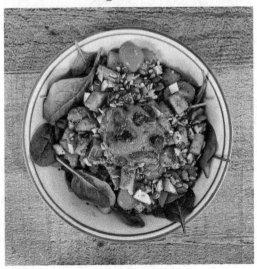

25. Potato Latke

Preparation Time: 15 minutes

Cooking Time: 10 minutes

Servings: 6

Ingredients:

3 eggs, beaten

1 onion, grated

1 ½ teaspoons baking powder

Salt and pepper to taste

2 lb. potatoes, peeled and grated

¼ cup all-purpose flour

4 tablespoons vegetable oil

Chopped onion chives

Direction

Preheat your oven to 400 degrees F.

In a bowl, beat the eggs, onion, baking powder, salt and pepper.

Squeeze moisture from the shredded potatoes using paper towel.

Add potatoes to the egg mixture.

Stir in the flour.

Pour the oil into a pan over medium heat.

Cook a small amount of the batter for 3 to 4 minutes per side.

Repeat until the rest of the batter is used.

Garnish with the chives.

Nutrition: Calories: 266 Total fat: 11.6g Saturated fat: 2g Cholesterol: 93mg Sodium: 360mg Potassium: 752mg Carbohydrates: 34.6g Fiber: 9g Sugar: 3g Protein: 7.5g

26. Broccoli Rabe

Preparation Time: 15 minutes

Cooking Time: 15 minutes

Servings: 8

Ingredients:

2 oranges, sliced in half

1 lb. broccoli rabe

2 tablespoons sesame oil, toasted

Salt and pepper to taste

1 tablespoon sesame seeds, toasted

Direction

Pour the oil into a pan over medium heat.

Add the oranges and cook until caramelized.

Transfer to a plate.

Put the broccoli in the pan and cook for 8 minutes.

Squeeze the oranges to release juice in a bowl.

Stir in the oil, salt and pepper.

Coat the broccoli rabe with the mixture.

Sprinkle seeds on top.

Nutrition: Calories: 59 Total fat: 4.4g Saturated fat: 0.6g Sodium: 164mg Potassium: 160mg Carbohydrates: 4.1g Fiber: 1.6g Sugar: 2g Protein: 2.2g

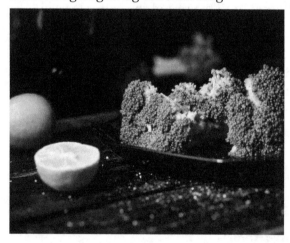

27. Whipped Potatoes

Preparation Time: 20 minutes

Cooking Time: 35 minutes

Servings: 10

Ingredients:

4 cups water

3 lb. potatoes, sliced into cubes

3 cloves garlic, crushed

6 tablespoons vegan butter

2 bay leaves

10 sage leaves

½ cup Vegan yogurt

¼ cup low-fat milk

Salt to taste

Direction

Boil the potatoes in water for 30 minutes or until tender.

Drain.

In a pan over medium heat, cook the garlic in butter for 1 minute.

Add the sage and cook for 5 more minutes.

Discard the garlic.

Use a fork to mash the potatoes.

Whip using an electric mixer while gradually adding the butter, yogurt, and milk.

Season with salt.

Nutrition: Calories: 169 Total fat: 7.6g Saturated fat: 4.7g Cholesterol: 21mg Sodium: 251mg Potassium: 519mg Carbohydrates: 22.1g Fiber: 1.5g Sugar: 2g Protein: 4.2g

28.   Quinoa Avocado Salad

Preparation Time: 15 minutes

Cooking Time: 4 minutes

Servings: 4

Ingredients:

2 tablespoons balsamic vinegar

¼ cup cream

¼ cup buttermilk

5 tablespoons freshly squeezed lemon juice, divided

1 clove garlic, grated

2 tablespoons shallot, minced

Salt and pepper to taste

2 tablespoons avocado oil, divided

1 ¼ cups quinoa, cooked

2 heads endive, sliced

2 firm pears, sliced thinly

2 avocados, sliced

¼ cup fresh dill, chopped

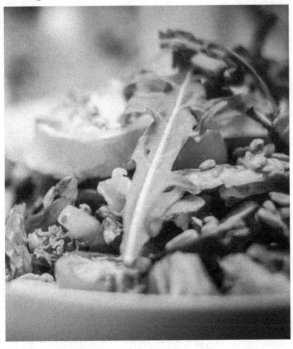

Direction

Combine the vinegar, cream, milk, 1 tablespoon lemon juice, garlic, shallot, salt and pepper in a bowl.

Pour 1 tablespoon oil into a pan over medium heat.

Heat the quinoa for 4 minutes.

Transfer quinoa to a plate.

Toss the endive and pears in a mixture of remaining oil, remaining lemon juice, salt and pepper.

Transfer to a plate.

Toss the avocado in the reserved dressing.

Add to the plate.

Top with the dill and quinoa.

Nutrition: Calories: 431 Total fat: 28.5g Saturated fat: 8g Cholesterol: 13mg Sodium: 345mg Potassium: 779mg Carbohydrates: 42.7g Fiber: 6g Sugar: 3g Protein: 6.6g

29.   Roasted Sweet Potatoes

Preparation Time: 20 minutes

Cooking Time: 20 minutes

Servings: 4

Ingredients:

2 potatoes, sliced into wedges

2 tablespoons olive oil, divided

Salt and pepper to taste

1 red bell pepper, chopped

¼ cup fresh cilantro, chopped

1 garlic, minced

2 tablespoons almonds, toasted and sliced

1 tablespoon lime juice

Direction

Preheat your oven to 425 degrees F.

Toss the sweet potatoes in oil and salt.

Transfer to a baking pan.

Roast for 20 minutes.

In a bowl, combine the red bell pepper, cilantro, garlic and almonds.

In another bowl, mix the lime juice, remaining oil, salt and pepper.

Drizzle this mixture over the red bell pepper mixture.

Serve sweet potatoes with the red bell pepper mixture.

Nutrition: Calories: 146 Total fat: 8.6g Saturated fat: 1.1g Sodium: 317mg Potassium: 380mg Carbohydrates: 16g Fiber: 2.9g Sugar: 5g Protein: 2.3g

30.   Cauliflower Salad

Preparation Time: 20 minutes

Cooking Time: 15 minutes

Servings: 4

Ingredients:

8 cups cauliflower florets

5 tablespoons olive oil, divided

Salt and pepper to taste

1 cup parsley

1 clove garlic, minced

2 tablespoons lemon juice

¼ cup almonds, toasted and sliced

3 cups arugula

2 tablespoons olives, sliced

¼ cup feta, crumbled

Direction

Preheat your oven to 425 degrees F.

Toss the cauliflower in a mixture of 1 tablespoon olive oil, salt and pepper.

Place in a baking pan and roast for 15 minutes.

Put the parsley, remaining oil, garlic, lemon juice, salt and pepper in a blender.

Pulse until smooth.

Place the roasted cauliflower in a salad bowl.

Stir in the rest of the ingredients along with the parsley dressing.

Nutrition: Calories: 198 Total fat: 16.5g Saturated fat: 3g Cholesterol: 6mg Sodium: 3mg Potassium: 570mg Carbohydrates: 10.4g Fiber: 4.1g Sugar: 4g Protein: 5.4g

31.   Garlic Mashed Potatoes & Turnips

Preparation Time: 20 minutes

Cooking Time: 30 minutes

Servings: 8

Ingredients:

1 head garlic

1 teaspoon olive oil

1 lb. turnips, sliced into cubes

2 lb. potatoes, sliced into cubes

½ cup almond milk

½ cup vegan parmesan cheese, grated

1 tablespoon fresh thyme, chopped

1 tablespoon fresh chives, chopped

2 tablespoons vegan butter

Salt and pepper to taste

Direction

Preheat your oven to 375 degrees F.

Slice the tip off the garlic head.

Drizzle with a little oil and roast in the oven for 45 minutes.

Boil the turnips and potatoes in a pot of water for 30 minutes or until tender.

Add all the ingredients to a food processor along with the garlic.

Pulse until smooth.

Nutrition: Calories: 141 Total fat: 3.2g Saturated fat: 1.5g Cholesterol: 7mg Sodium: 284mg Potassium: 676mg Carbohydrates: 24.6g Fiber: 3.1g Sugar: 4g Protein: 4.6g

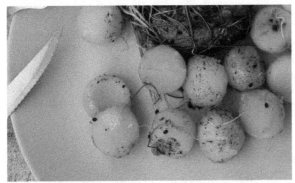

32. Green Beans with vegan Bacon

Preparation Time: 15 minutes

Cooking Time: 20 minutes

Servings: 8

Ingredients:

2 slices of vegan bacon, chopped

1 shallot, chopped

24 oz. green beans

Salt and pepper to taste

½ teaspoon smoked paprika

1 teaspoon lemon juice

2 teaspoons vinegar

Direction

Preheat your oven to 450 degrees F.

Add the bacon in the baking pan and roast for 5 minutes.

Stir in the shallot and beans.

Season with salt, pepper and paprika.

Roast for 10 minutes.

Drizzle with the lemon juice and vinegar.

Roast for another 2 minutes.

Nutrition: Calories: 49 Total fat: 1.2g Saturated fat: 0.4g Cholesterol: 3mg Sodium: 192mg Potassium: 249mg Carbohydrates: 8.1g Fiber: 3g Sugar: 4g Protein: 2.9g

33. Coconut Brussels Sprouts

Preparation Time: 15 minutes

Cooking Time: 10 minutes

Servings: 4

Ingredients:

1 lb. Brussels sprouts, trimmed and sliced in half

2 tablespoons coconut oil

¼ cup coconut water

1 tablespoon soy sauce

Direction

In a pan over medium heat, add the coconut oil and cook the Brussels sprouts for 4 minutes.

Pour in the coconut water.

Cook for 3 minutes.

Add the soy sauce and cook for another 1 minute.

Nutrition: Calories: 114 Total fat: 7.1g Saturated fat: 5.7g Sodium: 269mg Potassium: 483mg Carbohydrates: 11.1g Fiber: 4.3g Sugar: 3g Protein: 4g

34. Cod Stew with Rice & Sweet Potatoes

Preparation Time: 30 minutes

Cooking Time: 1 hour

Servings: 4

Ingredients:

2 cups water

¾ cup brown rice

1 tablespoon vegetable oil

1 tablespoon ginger, chopped

1 tablespoon garlic, chopped

1 sweet potato, sliced into cubes

1 bell pepper, sliced

1 tablespoon curry powder

Salt to taste

15 oz. coconut milk

4 cod fillets

2 teaspoons freshly squeezed lime juice

3 tablespoons cilantro, chopped

Direction

Place the water and rice in a saucepan.

Bring to a boil and then simmer for 30 to 40 minutes. Set aside.

Pour the oil in a pan over medium heat.

Cook the garlic for 30 seconds.

Add the sweet potatoes and bell pepper.

Season with curry powder and salt.

Mix well.

Pour in the coconut milk.

Simmer for 15 minutes.

Nestle the fish into the sauce and cook for another 10 minutes.

Stir in the lime juice and cilantro.

Serve with the rice.

Nutrition: Calories: 382 Total fat: 11.3g Saturated fat: 4.8g Cholesterol: 45mg Sodium: 413mg Potassium: 736mg Carbohydrates: 49.5g Fiber: 5.3g Sugar: 8g Protein: 19.2g

35. Vegan Chicken & Rice

Preparation Time: 15 minutes

Cooking Time: 3 hours and 30 minutes

Servings: 8

Ingredients:

8 Tofu thighs

Salt and pepper to taste

½ teaspoon ground coriander

2 teaspoons ground cumin

17 oz. brown rice, cooked

30 oz. black beans

1 tablespoon olive oil

Pinch cayenne pepper

2 cups pico de gallo

¾ cup radish, sliced thinly

2 avocados, sliced

Direction

Season the tofu with salt, pepper, coriander and cumin.

Place in a slow cooker.

Pour in the stock.

Cook on low for 3 hours and 30 minutes.

Place the tofu in a cutting board.

Shred the chicken.

Toss the tofu shreds in the cooking liquid.

Serve the rice in bowls, topped with the tofu and the rest of the ingredients.

Nutrition: Calories: 470 Total fat: 17g Saturated fat: 3g Sodium: 615mg Carbohydrates: 40g Fiber: 11g Sugar: 1g Protein: 40g

36.   Rice Bowl with Edamame

Preparation Time: 10 minutes

Cooking Time: 3 hours and 50 minutes

Servings: 6

Ingredients:

1 tablespoon coconut oil, melted

¾ cup brown rice (uncooked)

1 cup wild rice (uncooked)

Cooking spray

4 cups vegetable stock

8 oz. shelled edamame

1 onion, chopped

Salt to taste

½ cup dried cherries, sliced

½ cup pecans, toasted and sliced

1 tablespoon red wine vinegar

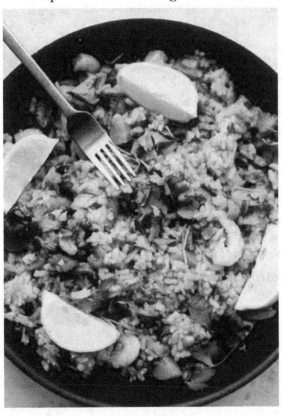

Direction

Add the rice and coconut oil in a slow cooker sprayed with oil.

Pour in the stock and stir in the edamame and onions.

Season with salt.

Seal the pot.

Cook on high for 3 hours and 30 minutes.

Stir in the dried cherries.

Let sit for 5 minutes.

Stir in the rest of the ingredients before serving.

Nutrition: Calories: 381 Total fat: 12g 18 % Saturated fat: 2g Sodium: 459mg Carbohydrates: 61g Fiber: 7g Sugar: 13g Protein: 12g

37.   Chickpea Avocado Sandwich

You can make the chickpea and avocado filling ahead of time and store it in the cold-storage box for or in the icebox. While avocado does brown easily, the lime juice helps preserve the integrity of it.

Preparation time: 10 minutes

Cooking Time: 5 minutes

Servings: 2

Ingredients:

Chickpeas – 1 can

Avocado – 1

Dill, dried – .25 teaspoon

Onion powder – .25 teaspoon

Sea salt – .5 teaspoon

Celery, chopped – .25 cup

Green onion, chopped – .25 cup

Lime juice – 3 tablespoons

Garlic powder – .5 teaspoon

Dark pepper, ground – dash

Tomato, sliced – 1

Lettuce – 4 leaves

Bread – 4 slices

Directions:

Drain the canned chickpeas and rinse them under cool water. Place them in a bowl along with the herbs, spices, sea salt, avocado, and lime juice. Using a potato masher or fork, mash the avocado and chickpeas together until you have a thick filling. Try not to mash the chickpeas all the way, as they create texture.

Stir the celery and green onion into the filling and prepare your sandwiches.

Layout two slices of bread, top them with the chickpea filling, some lettuce, and sliced tomato. Top them off with the two remaining slices, slice the sandwiches in half, and serve.

Nutrition: Calories 471

38.   Roasted Tomato Sandwich

This sandwich is full of fresh ingredients, many of which cannot be prepared ahead. But, when you simply have to prepare some lettuce, an avocado, or tomato, this is not a problem. You can still have an easy and quick meal. But, that doesn't mean you can't prepare any aspects of this sandwich ahead of time. If using homemade bread, you can prepare it at the beginning of the week and store it in the cold-storage box or icebox. You can also prepare the garlic aioli ahead of time and store it in a Mason jar in the fridge.

Preparation time: 30 minutes

Cooking Time: 25 minutes

Servings: 2

Ingredients:

Sourdough bread – 4 slices

Tomatoes, large, cut into eight rounds – 2

Avocado – 1

Sea salt – .25 teaspoon

Vegan mayonnaise – .25 cup

Garlic, minced – 2 cloves

Juice of lemon fruit – 1 tablespoon

Oregano, dried – .25 teaspoon

Black ground pepper – .25 teaspoon

Olive oil – 2 tablespoons

Fresh basil – .25 cup

Arugula – .25 cup

Directions:

Begin by setting your electric cooker to Fahrenheit 350 degrees and lining an aluminum sheet pan with kitchen parchment. Layout the sliced tomatoes on the sheet, and sprinkle them with part of the salt, oregano, and pepper, and allow them to roast until tender, about fifteen minutes.

Meanwhile, prepare the garlic aioli. Whisk together the mayonnaise, garlic, juice of lemon fruit, and some sea salt and pepper. Chill in the fridge until use.

Use a pastry brush and coat one side of each slice of bread with the olive oil. While doing this preheat a skillet over midway warmth. Once hot, toast the bread oil-side down until browned and then remove them from the heat.

To prepare the sandwiches, lay out the bread, oil side down. On each slice spread the garlic aioli. On half of the slices cover with the roasted tomatoes, sliced avocado, basil, and arugula. Top these slices with their matched slice without toppings. Slice the sandwiches in half before serving.

Nutrition: Calories 525

39.   Pulled "Pork" Sandwiches

This pulled "pork" is the perfect dish to make ahead. Prepare the mushrooms and coat them in the sauce and then you can store them chilled in the cold-storage box or the icebox. If you prepare a large amount to keep in the icebox, you will always have some on hand for sandwiches, pizza, nachos, or any other vegan-version of popular dishes that might be complemented by pulled "pork".

Preparation time: 40 minutes

Cooking Time: 35 minutes

Servings: 3

Ingredients:

King oyster mushrooms* – 4

Barbecue sauce – .25 cup

Olive oil – 2 tablespoons

Sea salt – .25 teaspoon

Garlic, minced – 2 cloves

Cayenne pepper – .25 teaspoon

Bread – 6 slices

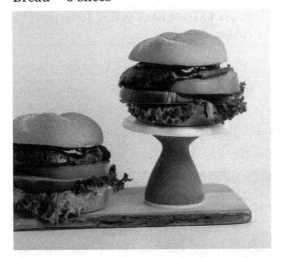

Directions:

Start by setting your electric cooker to Fahrenheit 400 degrees.

While your electric cooker warms up, clean the mushrooms with a damp paper towel and then use two forks to shred both the caps and stems of the mushrooms into pieces resembling pulled pork. Place the shredded mushrooms on a kitchen parchment-lined aluminum baking sheet.

Drizzle the mushrooms with half of the olive oil and then toss them with the seasoning and garlic until evenly coated. Allow the oyster mushrooms to roast until slightly crispy and browned about twenty minutes.

In a skillet, add the remaining tablespoon of olive oil, allowing it to warm over midway-elevated. Put the cooked mushrooms in the pan along with the barbecue sauce.

Cook the mushrooms in the sauce while stirring until the sauce is fragrant and warm, about three to five minutes. Top three slices of bread with this concoction and top with the remaining three slices. Cut the sandwiches in half before serving.

Note:

*If you can't find king oyster mushrooms, then you can use three heaping cups of regular oyster mushrooms.

Nutrition: Calories 259

Chapter 6: Recipes for Main Courses and Single Dishes

40. Noodles Alfredo with Herby Tofu

Preparation Time: 10 minutes

Cooking Time: 5 minutes

Servings: 4

Ingredients:

2 tbsp vegetable oil

2 (14 oz.) blocks extra-firm tofu, pressed and cubed

12 ounces eggless noodles

1 tbsp dried mixed herbs

2 cups cashews, soaked overnight and drained

¾ cups unsweetened almond milk

½ cup nutritional yeast

4 garlic cloves, roasted (roasting is optional but highly recommended)

½ cup onion, coarsely chopped

1 lemon, juiced

½ cup sun-dried tomatoes

Salt and black pepper to taste

2 tbsp chopped fresh basil leaves to garnish

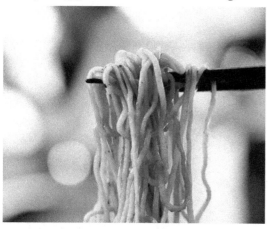

Directions:

Heat the vegetable oil in a large skillet over medium heat.

Season the tofu with the mixed herbs, salt, black pepper, and fry in the oil until golden brown. Transfer to a paper-towel-lined plate and set aside. Turn the heat off.

In a blender, combine the almond milk, nutritional yeast, garlic, onion, and lemon juice. Set aside.

Reheat the vegetable oil in the skillet over medium heat and sauté the noodles for 2 minutes. Stir in the sundried tomatoes and the cashew (Alfredo) sauce. Reduce the heat to low and cook for 2 more minutes.

If the sauce is too thick, thin with some more almond milk to your desired thickness.

Dish the food, garnish with the basil and serve warm.

41. Lemon Couscous with Tempeh Kabobs

Preparation Time: 2 hours 15 minutes

Cooking Time: 2 hours

Servings: 4

Ingredients:

For the tempeh kabobs:

1 ½ cups of water

10 oz. tempeh, cut into 1-inch chunks

1 red onion, cut into 1-inch chunks

1 small yellow squash, cut into 1-inch chunks

1 small green squash, cut into 1-inch chunks

2 tbsp. olive oil

1 cup sugar-free barbecue sauce

8 wooden skewers, soaked

For the lemon couscous:

1 ½ cups whole wheat couscous

2 cups of water

Salt to taste

¼ cup chopped parsley

¼ chopped mint leaves

¼ cup chopped cilantro

1 lemon, juiced

1 medium avocado, pitted, sliced and peeled

Directions:

For the tempeh kabobs:

Boil the water in a medium pot over medium heat.

Once boiled, turn the heat off, and put the tempeh in it. Cover the lid and let the tempeh steam for 5 minutes (this is to remove its bitterness). Drain the tempeh after.

After, pour the barbecue sauce into a medium bowl, add the tempeh, and coat well with the sauce. Cover the bowl with plastic wrap and marinate for 2 hours.

After 2 hours, preheat a grill to 350 F.

On the skewers, alternately thread single chunks of the tempeh, onion, yellow squash, and green squash until the ingredients are exhausted.

Lightly grease the grill grates with olive oil, place the skewers on top and brush with some barbecue sauce. Cook for 3 minutes on each side while brushing with more barbecue sauce as you turn the kabobs.

Transfer to a plate for serving.

For the lemon couscous:

Meanwhile, as the kabobs cooked, pour the couscous, water, and salt into a medium bowl and steam in the microwave for 3 to 4 minutes. Remove the bowl from the microwave and allow slight cooling.

Stir in the parsley, mint leaves, cilantro, and lemon juice.

Garnish the couscous with the avocado slices and serve with the tempeh kabobs.

42.   Portobello Burger with Veggie Fries

Preparation Time: 45 minutes

Cooking Time: 30 minutes

Servings: 4

Ingredients:

For the veggie fries:

3 carrots, peeled and julienned

2 sweet potatoes, peeled and julienned

1 rutabaga, peeled and julienned

2 tsp olive oil

¼ tsp paprika

Salt and black pepper to taste

For the Portobello burgers:

1 clove garlic, minced

½ tsp salt

2 tbsp. olive oil

4 whole-wheat buns

4 Portobello mushroom caps

½ cup sliced roasted red peppers

2 tbsp. pitted Kalamata olives, chopped

2 medium tomatoes, chopped

½ tsp dried oregano

¼ cup crumbled feta cheese (optional)

1 tbsp. red wine vinegar

2 cups baby salad greens

½ cup hummus for serving

Directions:

For the veggie fries:

Preheat the oven to 400 F.

Spread the carrots, sweet potatoes, and rutabaga on a baking sheet and season with the olive oil, paprika, salt, and black pepper. Use your hands to rub the seasoning well onto the vegetables. Bake in the oven for 20 minutes or until the vegetables soften (stir halfway).

When ready, transfer to a plate and use it for serving.

For the Portobello burgers:

Meanwhile, as the vegetable roast, heat a grill pan over medium heat.

Use a spoon to crush the garlic with salt in a bowl. Stir in 1 tablespoon of the olive oil.

Brush the mushrooms on both sides with the garlic mixture and grill in the pan on both sides until tender, 8 minutes. Transfer to a plate and set aside.

Toast the buns in the pan until crispy, 2 minutes. Set aside in a plate.

In a bowl, combine the remaining ingredients except for the hummus and divide on the bottom parts of the buns.

Top with the hummus, cover the burger with the top parts of the buns and serve with the veggie fries.

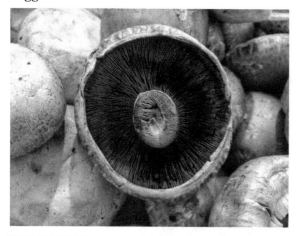

43.   Thai Seitan Vegetable Curry

Preparation Time: 20 minutes

Cooking Time: 15 minutes

Servings: 4

 Ingredients:

1 tbsp vegetable oil

4 cups diced seitan

1 cup sliced mixed bell peppers

½ cup onions diced

1 small head broccoli, cut into florets

2 tbsp Thai red curry paste

1 tsp garlic puree

1 cup unsweetened coconut milk

2 tbsp vegetable broth

2 cups spinach

Salt and black pepper to taste

Directions:

Heat the vegetable oil in a large skillet over medium heat and fry the seitan until slightly dark brown. Mix in the bell peppers, onions, broccoli, and cook until softened, 4 minutes.

Mix the curry paste, garlic puree, and 1 tablespoon of coconut milk. Cook for 1 minute and stir in the remaining coconut milk and vegetable broth. Simmer for 10 minutes.

Stir in the spinach to wilt and season the curry with salt and black pepper.

Serve the curry with steamed white or brown rice.

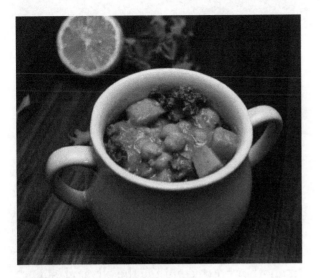

44.   Tofu Cabbage Stir-Fry

Preparation Time: 15 minutes

Cooking Time: 10 minutes

Servings: 4

Ingredients:

5 oz. vegan butter

2 ½ cups baby bok choy, quartered lengthwise

8 oz sliced mushrooms

2 cups extra-firm tofu, pressed and cubed

Salt and black pepper to taste

1 tsp onion powder

1 tsp garlic powder

1 tbsp plain vinegar

2 garlic cloves, minced

1 tsp chili flakes

1 tbsp fresh ginger, grated

3 scallions, sliced

1 tbsp sesame oil

1 cup vegan mayonnaise

Wasabi paste to taste

Cooked white or brown rice (1/2 cup per person)

Directions:

Melt half of the vegan butter in a wok and sauté the bok choy until softened, 3 minutes.

Season with salt, black pepper, onion powder, garlic powder, and vinegar. Sauté for 2 minutes to combine the flavors and plate the bok choy.

Melt the remaining vegan butter in the wok and sauté the garlic, mushrooms, chili flakes, and ginger until fragrant.

Stir in the tofu and cook until browned on all sides. Add the scallions and bok choy, heat for 2 minutes and drizzle in the sesame oil.

In a small bowl, mix the vegan mayonnaise and wasabi, and mix into the tofu and vegetables. Cook for 2 minutes and dish the food.

Serve warm with steamed rice.

45.   Curried Tofu with Buttery Cabbage

Preparation Time: 15 minutes

Cooking Time: 10 minutes

Servings: 4

Ingredients:

2 cups extra-firm tofu, pressed and cubed

1 tbsp + 3 ½ tbsp coconut oil

½ cup unsweetened shredded coconut

1 tsp yellow curry powder

1 tsp salt

½ tsp onion powder

2 cups Napa cabbage

4 oz. vegan butter

Salt and black pepper to taste

Lemon wedges for serving

Directions:

In a medium bowl, add the tofu, 1 tablespoon of coconut oil, curry powder, salt, and onion powder. Mix well until the tofu is well-coated with the spices.

Heat the remaining coconut oil in a non-stick skillet and fry the tofu until golden brown on all sides, 8 minutes. Divide onto serving plates and set aside for serving.

In another skillet, melt half of the vegan butter, and sauté the cabbage until slightly caramelized, 2 minutes. Season with salt, black pepper, and plate to the side of the tofu.

Melt the remaining vegan butter in the skillet and drizzle all over the cabbage.

Serve warm.

46. Smoked Tempeh with Broccoli Fritters

Preparation Time: 25 minutes

Cooking Time: 20 minutes

Servings: 4

Ingredients:

For the flax egg:

4 tbsp flax seed powder + 12 tbsp water

For the grilled tempeh:

3 tbsp olive oil

1 tbsp soy sauce

3 tbsp fresh lime juice

1 tbsp grated ginger

Salt and cayenne pepper to taste

10 oz. tempeh slices

For the broccoli fritters:

2 cups of rice broccoli

8 oz. tofu cheese

3 tbsp plain flour

½ tsp onion powder

1 tsp salt

¼ tsp freshly ground black pepper

4¼ oz. vegan butter

For serving:

½ cup mixed salad greens

1 cup vegan mayonnaise

½ lemon, juiced

Directions:

For the smoked tempeh:

In a bowl, mix the flax seed powder with water and set aside to soak for 5 minutes.

In another bowl, combine the olive oil, soy sauce, lime juice, grated ginger, salt, and cayenne pepper. Brush the tempeh slices with the mixture.

Heat a grill pan over medium heat and grill the tempeh on both sides until nicely smoked and golden brown, 8 minutes. Transfer to a plate and set aside in a warmer for serving.

In a medium bowl, combine the broccoli rice, tofu cheese, flour, onion, salt, and black pepper. Mix in the flax egg until well combine and form 1-inch thick patties out of the mixture.

Melt the vegan butter in a medium skillet over medium heat and fry the patties on both sides until golden brown, 8 minutes. Remove the fritters onto a plate and set aside.

In a small bowl, mix the vegan mayonnaise with the lemon juice.

Divide the smoked tempeh and broccoli fritters onto serving plates, add the salad greens, and serve with the vegan mayonnaise sauce.

47. Cheesy Potato Casserole

Preparation Time: 30 minutes

Cooking Time: 20 minutes

Servings: 4

Ingredients:

2 oz. vegan butter

½ cup celery stalks, finely chopped

1 white onion, finely chopped

1 green bell pepper, seeded and finely chopped

Salt and black pepper to taste

2 cups peeled and chopped potatoes

1 cup vegan mayonnaise

4 oz. freshly shredded vegan Parmesan cheese

1 tsp red chili flakes

Directions:

Preheat the oven to 400 F and grease a baking dish with cooking spray.

Season the celery, onion, and bell pepper with salt and black pepper.

In a bowl, mix the potatoes, vegan mayonnaise, Parmesan cheese, and red chili flakes.

Pour the mixture into the baking dish, add the season vegetables, and mix well.

Bake in the oven until golden brown, about 20 minutes.

Remove the baked potato and serve warm with baby spinach.

48. Curry Mushroom Pie

Preparation Time: 65 minutes

Cooking Time: 1 hour

Servings: 4

Ingredients:

For the piecrust:

1 tbsp flax seed powder + 3 tbsp water

¾ cup plain flour

4 tbsp. chia seeds

4 tbsp almond flour

1 tbsp nutritional yeast

1 tsp baking powder

1 pinch salt

3 tbsp olive oil

4 tbsp water

For the filling:

1 cup chopped baby Bella mushrooms

1 cup vegan mayonnaise

3 tbsp + 9 tbsp water

½ red bell pepper, finely chopped

1 tsp curry powder

½ tsp paprika powder

½ tsp garlic powder

¼ tsp black pepper

½ cup coconut cream

1¼ cups shredded vegan Parmesan cheese

Directions:

In two separate bowls, mix the different portions of flaxseed powder with the respective quantity of water. Allow soaking for 5 minutes.

For the piecrust:

Preheat the oven to 350 F.

When the flax egg is ready, pour the smaller quantity into a food processor and pour in all the ingredients for the piecrust. Blend until soft, smooth dough forms.

Line an 8-inch springform pan with parchment paper and grease with cooking spray.

Spread the dough in the bottom of the pan and bake for 15 minutes.

For the filling:

In a bowl, add the remaining flax egg and all the filling's ingredients. Combine well and pour the mixture on the piecrust. Bake further for 40 minutes or until the pie is golden brown.

Remove from the oven and allow cooling for 1 minute.

Slice and serve the pie warm.

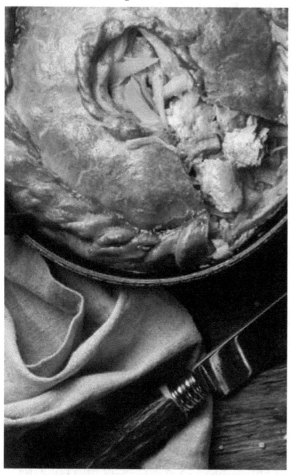

49.   Spicy Cheesy Tofu Balls

Preparation Time: 30 minutes

Cooking Time: 15 minutes

Servings: 4

Ingredients:

⅓ cup vegan mayonnaise

¼ cup pickled jalapenos

1 pinch cayenne pepper

4 oz. grated vegan cheddar cheese

1 tsp paprika powder

1 tbsp mustard powder

1 tbsp flax seed powder + 3 tbsp water

2 ½ cup crumbled tofu

Salt and black pepper to taste

2 tbsp vegan butter, for frying

Directions:

For the spicy cheese:

In a bowl, mix all the ingredients for the spicy vegan cheese until well combined. Set aside.

In another medium bowl, combine the flax seed powder with water and allow soaking for 5 minutes.

Add the flax egg to the cheese mixture, the crumbled tofu, salt, and black pepper, and combine well. Use your hands to form large meatballs out of the mix.

Melt the vegan butter in a large skillet over medium heat and fry the tofu balls until cooked and golden brown on all sides, 10 minutes.

Serve the tofu balls with your favorite mashes or in burgers.

50. Radish Chips

Preparation Time: 20 Minutes

Cooking Time: 10 Minutes

Servings: 4

Ingredients:

10-15 Radishes, Large

Sea Salt & Black Pepper to Taste

Directions:

Start by heating your oven to 375.

Slice your radishes thin, and then spread them out on a cookie sheet that's been sprayed with cooking spray.

Mist the radishes with cooking spray, and then season with salt and pepper.

Bake for ten minutes, and then flip.

Bake for five to ten minutes more. They should be crispy.

Interesting Facts: Potatoes are a great starchy source of potassium and protein. They are pretty inexpensive if you are one that is watching their budget. Bonus: Very heart healthy!

51. Sautéed Pears

Preparation Time: 35 Minutes

Cooking Time: 30 Minutes

Servings: 6

Ingredients:

2 Tablespoons Margarine (Or Vegan Butter)

¼ Teaspoon Cinnamon

¼ Teaspoon Nutmeg

6 Bosc Pears, Peeled & Quartered

1 Tablespoon Lemon Juice

½ Cup Walnuts, Toasted & Chopped (Optional)

Directions:

Melt your vegan butter in a skillet, and then add your spices. Cook for a half a minute before adding in your pears.

Cook for fifteen minutes, and then stir in your lemon juice.

Serve with walnuts if desired.

Interesting Facts: Cinnamon: This spice is an absolute powerhouse and is considered one of the healthiest, beneficial spices on the plant. It's widely known for its medicinal properties. This spice is loaded with powerful antioxidants and is popular for its anti-inflammatory properties. It can reduce heart disease and lower blood sugar levels.

52. Pecan & Blueberry Crumble

Preparation Time: 40 Minutes

Cooking Time: 1 Hour

Servings: 6

Calories: 381

Protein: 10 Grams

Fat: 32 Grams

Net Carbs: 20 Grams

Ingredients:

14 Ounces Blueberries

1 Tablespoon Lemon Juice, Fresh

1 ½ Teaspoon Stevia Powder

3 Tablespoons Chia Seeds

2 Cups Almond Flour, Blanched

¼ Cup Pecans, Chopped

5 Tablespoon coconut Oil

2 Tablespoon Cinnamon

Directions:

Mix together your blueberries, stevia, chia seeds and lemon juice, and place it in an iron skillet.

Mix ingredients while spreading it over your

blueberries.

Heat your oven to 400, and then transfer it to an oven safe skillet, baking for a half hour.

Interesting Facts: Blueberries: These guys are a delectable treat that is easily incorporated into many dishes. They are packed with antioxidants and Vitamin C. Bonus: Blueberries have been proven to promote eye health and slow macular degeneration.

53. Rice Pudding

Preparation Time: 1 Hour 35 Minutes

Cooking Time: 1 Hour and 30 Minutes

Servings: 6

Ingredients:

1 Cup Brown Rice

1 Teaspoon Vanilla Extract, Pure

½ Teaspoon Sea Salt, Fine

½ Teaspoon Cinnamon

¼ Teaspoon Nutmeg

3 Egg Substitutes

3 Cups Coconut Milk, Light

2 Cups Brown Rice, Cooked

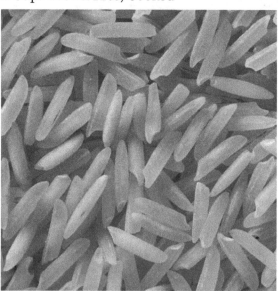

Directions:

Blend all of your ingredients together before pouring them into a two quarter dish.

Bake at 300 for ninety minutes before serving.

Interesting Facts: Brown rice is incredibly high in antioxidants and good vitamins. It's relative, 14 white rice is far less beneficial as much of these healthy nutrients get destroyed during the process of milling. You can also opt for red and black rice or wild rice. The meal options for this healthy grain are limitless!

54. Mango Sticky Rice

Preparation Time: 35 Minutes

Cooking Time: 30 Minutes

Servings: 3

Calories: 571

Protein: 6 Grams

Fat: 29.6 Grams

Carbs: 77.6 Grams

Ingredients:

½ Cup Sugar

1 Mango, Sliced

14 Ounces Coconut Milk, Canned

½ Cup Basmati Rice

Directions:

Cook your rice per package instructions, and add half of your sugar. When cooking your rice, substitute half of your water for half of your coconut milk.

Boil your remaining coconut milk in a saucepan with your remaining sugar.

Boil on high heat until it's thick, and then add in your mango slices.

Interesting Facts: Mangos contain 50% of the daily Vitamin C you should consume which aid in bone and immune health.

Chapter 7:   Snacks

55.   Beans with Sesame Hummus

Preparation time: 10 minutes

Cooking time: 0 minutes

Servings: 6

Ingredients

4 Tbsp sesame oil

2 cloves garlic finely sliced

1 can (15 oz) cannellini beans, drained

4 Tbsp sesame paste

2 Tbsp lemon juice freshly squeezed

1/4 tsp red pepper flakes

2 Tbsp fresh basil finely chopped

2 Tbsp fresh parsley finely chopped

Sea salt to taste

Directions:

Place all ingredients in your food processor.

Process until all ingredients are combined well and smooth.

Transfer mixture into a bowl and refrigerate until servings.

56.   Candied Honey-Coconut Peanuts

Preparation time: 15 minutes

Cooking time: 10 minutes

Servings: 8

Ingredients

1/2 cup honey (preferably a darker honey)

4 Tbsp coconut butter softened

1 tsp ground cinnamon

4 cups roasted, salted peanuts

Directions

Add honey, coconut butter, and cinnamon in a microwave-safe bowl.

Microwave at HIGH for about 4 to 5 minutes.

Stir in nuts; mix thoroughly to coat.

Microwave at HIGH 5 to 6 minutes or until foamy; stir after 3 minutes.

Spread in a single layer on a greased tray.

Refrigerated for 6 hours.

Break into small pieces and serve.

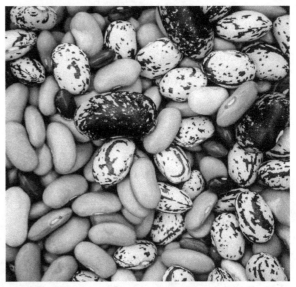

57. Choco Walnuts Fat Bombs

Preparation time: 15 minutes

Cooking time: 0 minutes

Servings: 6

Ingredients

1/2 cup coconut butter

1/2 cup coconut oil softened

4 Tbs cocoa powder, unsweetened

4 Tbs brown sugar firmly packed

1/3 cup silken tofu mashed

1 cup walnuts, roughly chopped

Directions

Add coconut butter and coconut oil into a microwave dish; melt it for 10-15 seconds.

Add in cocoa powder and whisk well.

Pour mixture into a blender with brown sugar and silken tofu cream; blend for 3-4 minutes.

Place silicone molds onto a sheet pan and fill halfway with chopped walnuts.

Pour the mixture over the walnuts and place it in the freezer for 6 hours.

Ready! Serve!

58. Crispy Honey Pecans (Slow Cooker)

Preparation time: 2 hours and 15 minutes

Cooking time: 3 hours

Servings: 4

Ingredients

16 oz pecan halves

4 Tbsp coconut butter melted

4 to 5 Tbsp honey strained

1/4 tsp ground ginger

1/4 tsp ground allspice

1 1/2 tsp ground cinnamon

Directions

Add pecans and melted coconut butter into your 4-quart Slow Cooker.

Stir until combined well.

Add in honey and stir well.

In a bowl, combine spices and sprinkle over nuts; stir lightly.

Cook on LOW uncovered for about 2 to 3 hours or until nuts are crispy.

Serve cold.

59. Crunchy Fried Pickles

Preparation time: 10 minutes

Cooking time: 5 minutes

Servings: 6

Ingredients

1/2 cup Vegetable oil for frying

1 cup all-purpose flour

1 cup plain breadcrumbs

Pinch of salt and pepper

30 pickle chips (cucumber, dill)

Directions:

Heat oil in a large frying skillet over medium-high heat.

Stir the flour, breadcrumbs, and the salt and pepper in a shallow bowl.

Dredge the pickles in the flour/breadcrumbs mixture to coat completely.

Fry in batches until golden brown on all sides, 2 to 3 minutes in total.

Drain on paper towels and serve.

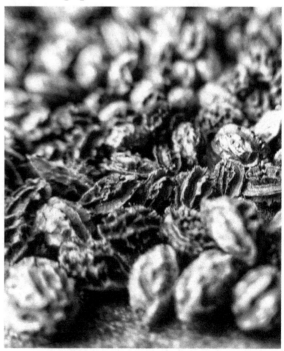

60.   Granola bars with Maple Syrup

Preparation time: 15 minutes

Cooking time: 0 minutes

Servings: 12

Ingredients

3/4 cup dates chopped

2 Tbsp chia seeds soaked

3/4 cup rolled oats

4 Tbsp Chopped nuts such Macadamia, almond, Brazilian...etc,

2 Tbsp shredded coconut

2 Tbsp pumpkin seeds

2 Tbsp sesame seeds

2 Tbsp hemp seeds

1/2 cup maple syrup (or to taste)

1/4 cup peanut butter

Directions:

Add all ingredients (except maple syrup and peanut butter) into a food processor and pulse just until roughly combined.

Add maple syrup and peanut butter and process until all ingredients are combined well.

Place baking paper onto a medium baking dish and spread the mixture.

Cover with a plastic wrap and press down to make it flat.

Chill granola in the fridge for one hour.

Cut it into 12 bars and serve.

Keep stored in an airtight container for up to 1 week.

Also, you can wrap them individually in parchment paper, and keep in the freezer in a large Ziploc bag.

61.Green Soy Beans Hummus

Preparation time: 15 minutes

Cooking time: 0 minutes

Servings: 6

Ingredients

1 1/2 cups frozen green soybeans

4 cups of water

coarse salt to taste

1/4 cup sesame paste

1/2 tsp grated lemon peel

3 Tbsp fresh lemon juice

2 cloves of garlic crushed

1/2 tsp ground cumin

1/4 tsp ground coriander

4 Tbsp extra virgin olive oil

1 Tbsp fresh parsley leaves chopped

Serving options: sliced cucumber, celery, olives

Directions:

1. In a saucepan, bring to boil 4 cups of water with 2 to 3 pinch of coarse salt.

2. Add in frozen soybeans, and cook for 5 minutes or until tender.

3. Rinse and drain soybeans into a colander.

4. Add soybeans and all remaining ingredients into a food processor.

5. Pulse until smooth and creamy.

6. Taste and adjust salt to taste.

7. Serve with sliced cucumber, celery, olives, bread...etc.

62. High Protein Avocado Guacamole

Preparation time: 15 minutes

Cooking time: 0 minutes

Servings: 4

Ingredients

1/2 cup of onion, finely chopped

1 chili pepper (peeled and finely chopped)

1 cup tomato, finely chopped

Cilantro leaves, fresh

2 avocados

2 Tbsp linseed oil

1/2 cup ground walnuts

1/2 lemon (or lime)

Salt

Directions:

Chop the onion, chili pepper, cilantro, and tomato; place in a large bowl.

Slice avocado, open vertically, and remove the pit.

Using the spoon take out the avocado flesh.

Mash the avocados with a fork and add into the bowl with onion mixture.

Add all remaining ingredients and stir well until ingredients combine well.

Taste and adjust salt and lemon/lime juice.

Keep refrigerated into covered glass bowl up to 5 days.

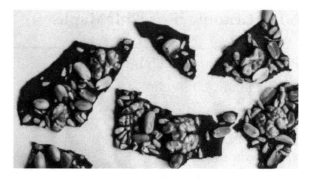

63. Homemade Energy Nut Bars

Preparation time: 15 minutes

Cooking time: 0 minutes

Servings: 4

Ingredients

1/2 cup peanuts

1 cup almonds

1/2 cup hazelnut, chopped

1 cup shredded coconut

1 cup almond butter

2 tsp sesame seeds toasted

1/2 cup coconut oil, freshly melted

2 Tbsp organic honey

1/4 tsp cinnamon

Directions

Add all nuts into a food processor and pulse for 1-2 minutes.

Add in shredded coconut, almond butter, sesame seeds, melted coconut oil, cinnamon, and honey; process only for one minute.

Cover a square plate/tray with parchment paper and apply the nut mixture.

Spread mixture vigorously with a spatula.

Place in the freezer for 4 hours or overnight.

Remove from the freezer and cut into rectangular bars.

Ready! Enjoy!

64.   Honey Peanut Butter

Preparation time: 10 minutes

Cooking time: 0 minutes

Servings: 6

Ingredients

1 cup peanut butter

3/4 cup honey extracted

1/2 cup ground peanuts

1 tsp ground cinnamon

Directions:

Add all ingredients into your fast-speed blender, and blend until smooth.

Keep refrigerated.

65.   Mediterranean Marinated Olives

Preparation time: 10 minutes

Cooking time: 0 minutes

Servings: 2

Ingredients

24 large olives, black, green, Kalamata

1/2 cup extra-virgin olive oil

4 cloves garlic, thinly sliced

2 Tbsp fresh lemon juice

2 tsp coriander seeds, crushed

1/2 tsp crushed red pepper

1 tsp dried thyme

1 tsp dried rosemary, crushed

Salt and ground pepper to taste

Directions:

Place olives and all remaining ingredients in a large container or bag, and shake to combine well.

Cover and refrigerate to marinate overnight.

Serve.

Keep refrigerated.

66.   Nut Butter & Dates Granola

Preparation time: 1 hour

Cooking time: 55 minutes

Servings: 8

Ingredients

3 cups rolled oats

2 cups dates, pitted and chopped

1 cup flaked or shredded coconut

1/2 cup wheat germ

1/4 cup soy milk powder

1/2 cup almonds chopped

3/4 cup honey strained

1/2 cup almond butter (plain, unsalted) softened

1/4 cup peanut butter softened

Directions:

Preheat oven to 300F.

Add all ingredients into a food processor and pulse until roughly combined.

Spread mixture evenly into greased 10 x 15-inch baking pan.

Bake for 45 to 55 minutes.

Stir mixture several times during baking.

Remove from the oven and cool completely.

Store in a covered glass jar.

67.   Oven-baked Caramelize Plantains

Preparation time: 30 minutes

Cooking time: 17 minutes

Servings: 4

Ingredients

4 medium plantains, peeled and sliced

2 Tbsp fresh orange juice

4 Tbsp brown sugar or to taste

1 Tbsp grated orange zest

4 Tbsp coconut butter, melted

Directions

Preheat oven to 360 F/180 C.

Place plantain slices in a heatproof dish.

Pour the orange juice over plantains, and then sprinkle with brown sugar and grated orange zest.

Melt coconut butter and pour evenly over plantains.

Cover with foil and bake for 15 to 17 minutes.

Serve warm or cold with honey or maple syrup.

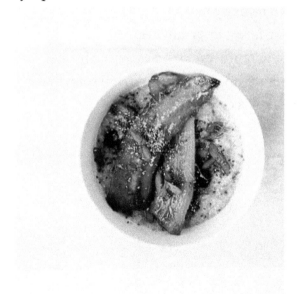

68.   Powerful Peas & Lentils Dip

Preparation time: 10 minutes

Cooking time: 0 minutes

Servings: 4

Ingredients

4 cups frozen peas

2 cup green lentils cooked

1 piece of grated ginger

1/2 cup fresh basil chopped

1 cup ground almonds

Juice of 1/2 lime

Pinch of salt

4 Tbsp sesame oil

1/4 cup Sesame seeds

Directions

Place all ingredients in a food processor or in a blender.

Blend until all ingredients combined well.

Keep refrigerated in an airtight container up to 4 days.

69.   Protein "Raffaello" Candies

Preparation time: 15 minutes

Cooking time: 0 minutes

Servings: 12

Ingredients

1 1/2 cups desiccated coconut flakes

1/2 cup coconut butter softened

4 Tbsp coconut milk canned

4 Tbs coconut palm sugar (or granulated sugar)

1 tsp pure vanilla extract

1 Tbsp vegan protein powder (pea or soy)

15 whole almonds

Directions

Put 1 cup of desiccated coconut flakes, and all remaining ingredients in the blender (except almonds), and blend until soft.

If your dough is too thick, add some coconut milk.

In a bowl, add remaining coconut flakes.

Coat every almond in one tablespoon of mixture and roll into a ball.

Roll each ball in coconut flakes.

Chill in the fridge for several hours.

70.   Protein-Rich Pumpkin Bowl

Preparation time: 10 minutes

Cooking time: 0 minutes

Servings: 2

Ingredients

1 1/2 cups almond milk (more or less depending on desired consistency)

1 cup pumpkin puree canned, with salt

1/2 cup chopped walnuts

1 scoop vegan soy protein powder

1 tsp pure vanilla extract

A handful of cacao nibs

Directions:

Add all ingredients in a blender apart from the cacao nibs.

Blend until smooth.

Serve in bowls and sprinkle with cacao nibs.

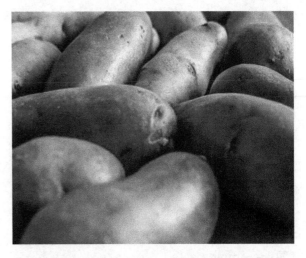

71. Savory Red Potato-Garlic Balls

Preparation time: 40 minutes

Cooking time: 25 minutes

Servings: 4

Ingredients

1 1/2 lbs of red potatoes

3 cloves of garlic finely chopped

1 Tbsp of fresh finely chopped parsley

1/4 tsp ground turmeric

Salt and ground pepper to taste

Directions:

Rinse potatoes and place unpeeled into a large pot.

Pour water to cover potatoes and bring to boil.

Cook for about 20 to 25 minutes on medium heat.

Rinse potatoes and let them cool down.

Peel potatoes and mash them; add finely chopped garlic, and the salt and pepper.

Form the potato mixture into small balls.

Sprinkle with chopped parsley and refrigerate for several hours.

Serve.

72. Spicy Smooth Red Lentil Dip

Preparation time: 35 minutes

Cooking time: 20 minutes

Servings: 4

Ingredients

1 cup red lentils

1 bay leaf

Sea salt to taste

2 garlic clove, finely chopped

2 Tbsp chopped cilantro leaves

1 Tbsp tomato paste

Lemon juice from 2 lemons, freshly squeezed

2 tsp ground cumin

4 Tbsp extra-virgin olive oil

Directions:

Rinse lentils and drain.

Combine lentils and bay leaf in a medium saucepan.

Pour enough water to cover lentils completely, and bring to boil.

Cover tightly, reduce heat to medium, and simmer for about 20 minutes.

Season salt to taste, and stir well. Note: Always season with the salt after cooking – if salt is added before, the lentils will become tough.

Drain the lentils in a colander. Discard the bay leaf and let the lentils cool for 10 minutes.

Transfer the lentils to a food processor and add all remaining ingredients.

Pulse until all ingredients combined well.

Taste and adjust seasonings if needed.

Transfer a lentil dip into a glass container and refrigerate at least 2 hours before serving.

73. Steamed Broccoli with Sesame

Preparation time: 15 minutes

Cooking time: 5 minutes

Servings: 2

Ingredients

1 1/2 lb fresh broccoli florets

1/2 cup sesame oil

4 Tbsp sesame seeds

Salt and ground pepper to taste

Directions:

Place broccoli florets in a steamer basket above boiling water.

Cover and steam for about 4 to 5 minutes.

Remove from steam and place broccoli in serving the dish.

Season with the salt and pepper, and drizzle with sesame oil; toss to coat.

Sprinkle with sesame seeds and serve immediately.

74. Vegan Eggplant Patties

Preparation time: 30 minutes

Cooking time: 15 minutes

Servings: 6

Ingredients

2 big eggplants

1 onion finely diced

1 Tbsp smashed garlic cloves

1 bunch raw parsley, chopped

1/2 cup almond meal

4 Tbsp Kalamata olives, pitted and sliced

1 Tbsp baking soda

Salt and ground pepper to taste

Olive oil or avocado oil, for frying

Directions

Peel off eggplants, rinse, and cut in half.

Sauté eggplant cubes in a non-stick skillet - occasionally stirring - about 10 minutes.

Transfer to a large bowl and mash with an immersion blender.

Add eggplant puree into a bowl and add in all remaining ingredients (except oil).

Knead a mixture using your hands until the dough is smooth, sticky, and easy to shape.

Shape mixture into 6 patties.

Heat the olive oil in a frying skillet on medium-high heat.

Fry patties for about 3 to 4 minutes per side.

Remove patties on a platter lined with kitchen paper towel to drain.

Serve warm.

75.Vegan Breakfast Sandwich

Preparation Time: 10minutes

Cooking Time: 10 minutes

Servings: 3

Ingredients

1 tsp. coconut oil

6 slices of bread

1 14 oz container

1-2 tsp. vegan extra firm tofu mayo

1 tsp. turmeric

1 cup of greens

1/2 tsp. garlic

1-2 medium powder tomatoes

1/2 tsp. Kala

6 pickle slices

Namak (black Fresh cracked salt) pepper

3 melty vegan cheese slices

Directions:

Season one facet of the tofu with salt, garlic powder, break up pepper, and turmeric. I just 15 sprinkled it out of the flavor bins. You will season the second side within the field when it is a perfect possibility to flip them.

In a medium skillet, warmth oil over medium warmth and notice the tofu cuts organized aspect down on the dish. While the bottom facet is cooking, season the pinnacle side. Let the tofu cook dinner for three to 5 minutes, till marginally darker and clean. Presently turn the cuts over and fry the alternative aspect for 3-5 minutes. Presently's a respectable time to pop the bread in the toaster, on every occasion liked.

To liquefy the cheddar, on a preparing sheet, place 2 cuts of tofu one next to the opposite, with a reduce of cheddar over every set. Put it within the broiler on prepare dinner for 1-three minutes, until the cheddar is dissolved. You can likewise utilize a toaster broiler.

Spread mayo on the two aspects of the bread.

Spot the two cuts of tofu with cheddar on one aspect. Include the vegetables and tomatoes.

Presently include several pickle cuts and near the sandwich collectively. Cut nook to corner

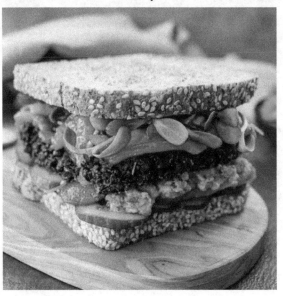

76. Chickpea And Mushroom Burger

Preparation Time: 20minutes

Cooking Time: 16 minutes

Serving: 4

Ingredients

240g chickpeas

Half tsp. sea salt

2 level tsp. gram

Half medium-flour

1 small red sized apple

1 tsp. dried onion

parsley

2 large cloves

1 tsp. fresh garlic

75g tasty rosemary

1 medium-sized mushrooms tomato

1 tsp. tahini

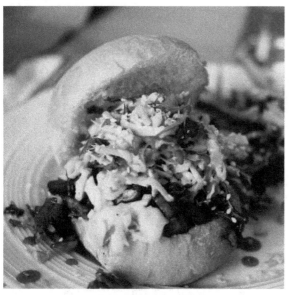

Directions

Pulverize garlic, diced onion and slash the mushrooms into little pieces; saute together in a search for a gold couple of moments.

Generally, pound chickpeas in an enormous blending bowl in with a potato masher or fork. The pound doesn't need to be absolutely smooth, in spite of the fact that you do need to give it a decent squeezing through with the goal that a great deal of it is very soft. It's fine to leave a couple of provincial looking pieces.

Mesh the half apple.

Include the gram flour, tahini, salt, and apple and combine all utilizing the rear of a metal spoon

Finely cleave the rosemary and slash the tomato into little pieces.

Include the sauteed things alongside every single residual ingredient into a bowl, pushing down and blending completely with a metal spoon.

Partition into 4 and solidly shape and form into patties.

Spot onto a barbecue plate and warmth under a medium flame broil for roughly 8 minutes on each side.

Chapter 8: Vegan Cheese

What is Vegan Cheese, and Why Are People going Nuts for it?

You may have seen some vegan cheeses in your local grocery stores and wonder, "Is it possible to make cheese without milk?"

With creative vegans trying to find an alternative to daily food items, countless cheese recipes have been done. There is now a wide selection of dairy-free cheeses in the market and recipes people enjoy.

Vegan cheese is a substitute for the conventional cheese people have grown eating. They're made with non-dairy or plant-based ingredients. Most consumers who buy and eat this type of cheese are vegan, but there are those who simply don't want to consume animal products for health reasons.

Vegan cheeses were first sold commercially in the 1980s. Back then, they weren't as popular as they are now. The first vegan cheeses sold usually tasted bad and had an obvious artificial texture.

Nowadays, vegan cheeses have evolved into something that can compete with commercial dairy cheeses. They taste better and have a texture closer to dairy cheese.

Many vegan cheeses use nuts as a base. They're packed with health benefits and contain fiber, minerals, and probiotics. There are also alternatives for people who have nut allergies.

One more thing that attracts people to consume vegan cheese is the wide array of vegan cheese recipes that are easy to do.

Different Types of Vegan Cheese Bases

Before trying any of the recipes in this book, you'll have to know the different bases of vegan cheese. This will help you determine what kind of vegan cheese you can make and enjoy at home.

Here are the ingredients used as a base for vegan cheese:

Seeds And Nuts

These are the most commonly used base for homemade vegan cheese.

Seeds and nuts are often soaked, processed, or fermented when used for making dairy-free cheeses. These ingredients taste bland on their own, meaning adding and combining flavors remains easy.

The nuts and seeds most often used for vegan cheese recipes are:

- Cashews

- Macadamia

- Almonds

- Sunflower seeds

- Pumpkin seeds

Soy

Commercial vegan cheeses are commonly soy-based. Soy products are used because they have the closest characteristics to real cheese.

Tofu may be the most widely used form of soy protein for vegan cheese. Both soft or silken and firm tofu can become different types of soft and hard cheeses. Tofu is blander than nuts, so achieving a cheese-like taste is definitely possible.

Soy is sometimes combined with a milk protein called casein. This protein allows the resulting cheese to have a melty characteristic, just like the real thing. But, to be perfectly clear, cheeses with casein aren't considered vegan.

What's a bit worrying though, is that some commercial cheeses labeled as vegan or vegetarian actually contain small amounts of the milk protein.

Flour

More often, flour is only a supplementary ingredient to other vegan cheese bases. But, there are some recipes that use flour as the base. Flour is usually used to create vegan cheese sauces though.

Some of the popular starchy flours used for vegan cheese recipes are:

- Tapioca starch/flour
- All-purpose flour
- Potato starch/flour
- Arrowroot flour

Vegetables

Some vegan cheeses have root vegetables as the base. The most common vegetables used are carrots and potatoes. Cheeses which use these as bases often have a soft and saucy consistency.

Non-Dairy Milk

Vegan cheese can also have non-dairy or plant-based milk as a base. It doesn't have casein like animal's milk, so vegan cheeses couldn't mimic the melty quality of real cheese. Other ingredients can be added, however, to somehow make the cruelty-free alternative a bit more similar.

Solidified Vegetable Oils

One of the things that people love about cheese is the creaminess. Some vegan cheeses use vegetable oils which are naturally loaded with fat, making it possible to copy the creaminess of real cheese. But, oils alone cannot serve as a base. Other ingredients like starch, flour, and agar-agar powder are used to create cheeses with vegetable oils.

77. Nut Milk

Seed-Free, Soy-Free

Making homemade Nut Milk is incredibly easy to do and yields a product far more delicious than buying it from the store. The process is the same for all nut and seed milks, but the soaking time varies. After you make Nut Milk a few times, it will be your new normal and set the foundation for so many other dairy-free recipes, especially vegan cheese!

Preparation time: 12 hours

Cooking time: 0 minutes

Servings: 4 to 6 cups

Active time: 12 minutes

Inactive Time: Varies, depending on nut soaking time

Ingredients

1 cup nuts (cashews, almonds, or walnuts)

4 to 6 cups filtered water

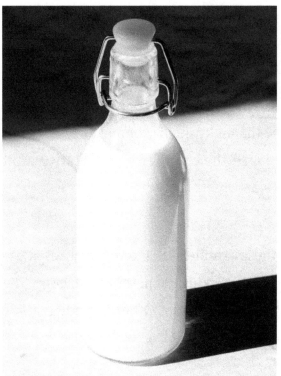

Directions:

In a small bowl, soak the nuts in water for the required time (8 to 12 hours for almonds or 6 to 12 hours for cashews and walnuts). Drain and rinse the nuts.

In a high-speed blender, combine the nuts with 4 to 6 cups of filtered water, depending on how creamy or thin you'd like the milk to be.

Blend for 2 minutes on high and then pour through a nut milk bag or cheesecloth set over a large pitcher. Squeeze out the liquid.

Storage: Place in an airtight container and refrigerate for 5 to 7 days.

Recipe Tip: For coffee creamer, I only add 4 cups of water, but for all of my other milk needs I add 6 cups of water to stretch the nuts as far as they can go.

If you want a flavored Nut Milk, try adding in a bit of any or all of the following: maple syrup, dates, sea salt, vanilla, cinnamon, or cocoa powder. Yum!

78. Hemp Milk

Nut-Free, Soy-Free

Hemp Milk is a great source of fiber, protein, and omega fatty acids that is nut-free! It tastes slightly earthy and has a great creamy consistency. The best part is that soaking is not required!

Preparation time: 10 minutes

Cooking time: 0 minutes

Servings: 2 pints

Ingredients

1 cup hemp hearts

4 cups filtered water

Directions:

In a high-speed blender, process the hemp hearts and water for 2 minutes.

Set cheesecloth or a nut milk bag over a pitcher, and pour the milk into it.

Storage: Place in an airtight container in the refrigerator for 5 to 7 days.

Recipe Tip: Because hemp hearts don't have skin, there really is no need to strain every time. But if you're going to be using Hemp Milk in another recipe application that requires a smooth final product, like most cheese, then I would still recommend it.

79.   Coconut Yogurt

Nut-Free, Seed-Free, Soy-Free

Coconut Yogurt became a staple in my kitchen shortly after its debut appearance. I was amazed at how simple it was—using just two ingredients—and how tangy it came out after the fermentation process. It can be used in so many preparations, and as you will find in this book, it can bring vegan cheese to the next level. Learn this recipe and your dairy-free horizons will expand.

Preparation time: 24 hours

Cooking time: 0 minutes

Servings: 1 pint

Active time: 12 minutes

Inactive Time: 24 hours to ferment, 20 minutes to chill

Ingredients

1 (13.6-ounce) can extra-rich coconut milk

1 Lactobacillus probiotic capsule

Directions:

In a glass jar, combine the coconut milk and the contents of the probiotic capsule, discarding the capsule. Stir with a wooden spoon to combine.

Top the lid with cheesecloth, about four layers thick, and secure with a string.

Leave at room temperature for 24 hours so the yogurt ferments.

Refrigerate for at least 20 minutes before serving.

Storage: Place the jar in the refrigerator for up to 5 days.

Recipe Tip: If a thick Greek-style yogurt is what you're looking for, scrape off the thicker coconut cream that forms at the top of the can to use and leave out the thin liquid at the bottom. In this case, you will need 2 cans to make the same amount of yogurt.

80.   Quinoa Rejuvelac

Nut-Free, Seed-Free, Soy-Free

Rejuvelac is a magical liquid that's created when you soak whole grains. The sprouting process creates a bit of fermentation in the water, and that water is what's used to flavor and further ferment many artisan vegan cheeses. You can also drink this on its own for probiotic health benefits. Using quinoa in this ferment produces a lemony, floral, and effervescent taste.

Preparation time: 3 days and 6 hours

Cooking time: 0 minutes

Servings: 1 pint

Active Time: 12 Minutes

Inactive Time: 3 To 4 Days

Ingredients

½ cup quinoa

Directions:

Rinse and drain the quinoa, and then place in a glass jar and cover with water by 1 inch. Cover with a cheesecloth and secure tightly with a string.

Leave overnight to sprout. If the grains don't sprout overnight, drain and rinse the quinoa, and let sit for another 4 to 6 hours, moist but not submerged in water.

Repeat the rinse a few times a day until the grains sprout.

Once the quinoa has sprouted, place it back in the glass jar and cover it with 2 cups of filtered water. Cover with cheesecloth and secure tightly with a string. Place in a cool dry place for 2 to 3 days until it develops a tangy flavor and smell. Strain the liquid from the quinoa, discarding (or reusing) the quinoa.

Storage: Place in an airtight container and refrigerate for up to 7 days.

Recipe Tip: You can make a second batch using the same quinoa and covering it with 2 cups of water again!

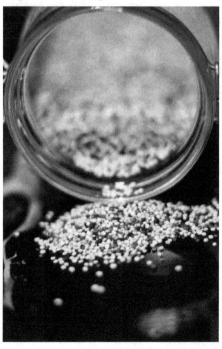

81.Barley Rejuvelac

Nut-Free, Seed-Free, Soy-Free

Using barley as the grain for rejuvelac produces a musky, earthy flavor that goes great in some of the richer, funkier cheeses.

Preparation time: 3 days and 6 hours

Cooking time: 0 minutes

Servings: 1 pint

Active Time: 12 minutes

Inactive Time: 3 to 4 days

Ingredients

½ cup barley

Directions:

Rinse and drain the barley, and then place in a glass jar and cover with water by 1 inch. Cover with a cheesecloth and secure tightly with a string.

Leave overnight to sprout. If the grains don't sprout overnight, drain the barley and let sit for another 4 to 6 hours, moist but not submerged in water.

Repeat the rinse a few times a day until the grains sprout.

Once the barley has sprouted, place it back in the glass jar and cover with 2 cups of filtered water. Cover with cheesecloth and secure tightly with a string. Place in a cool dry place for 2 to 3 days until it develops a tangy flavor and smell. Strain the liquid from the barley, discarding the barley.

Storage: Place in an airtight container and refrigerate for 7 days.

Recipe Tip: If white clouds appear on the surface of the liquid, scrape them off. This is not a bad thing, but if left unchecked, it can add bitterness to the final product.

Chapter 9:   Nutrient Deficiencies of a Vegan Diet (And How to Solve Them)

Now, one of the main drawbacks to a plant-based diet is that there are some nutrient deficiencies that you'll have to address. From an athletic performance and/or muscle building standpoint, understanding and addressing these concerns should be one of your highest priorities. These deficiencies come about because human beings are biologically designed to be omnivorous, i.e. to eat a mixture of plant and animal products. In choosing a wholly plant-based diet you will end up lacking a few nutrients that you would normally get from animal products, so you'll need to eat carefully or supplement to make up for this.

Vitamin B-12

Vitamin B-12 is a water-soluble vitamin, common sources of which include liver, clams, sardines, beef, tuna and a variety of other animal products. It is also one of the only nutrients that the human body cannot naturally produce for itself, so consuming adequate amounts is essential. Vitamin B-12 helps to maintain healthy nerves and brain function as well as support DNA and red blood cell production.

Deficiency can lead to a whole host of health problems including anaemia, ulcers, muscle weakness, extreme fatigue, depression, confusion and memory issues (Skerret 2013).

Now, since it's hard to perform at your athletic best when you're confused, weak and depressed, you're probably going to want to address this deficiency. Unfortunately, as there are no plant-based sources of B-12, you're going to have to eat certain fortified foods or supplements to address this. On the plus side the recommended daily intake (RDI) of B-12 is very achievable at around 2.4 mcg, with slightly higher amounts recommended for pregnant or breastfeeding women as well as people over the age of 65.

The simplest alternatives are fortified cereals, a standard cup of which contains over 140% of your RDI, and fortified milks, a standard cup of which contains around 45% of your RDI. When eaten together a bowl of fortified cereal with fortified milk will get you close to 200% of your recommended daily intake. If you're not a big fan of cereal or milk, you can also buy vitamin B-12 supplements for very reasonable prices (200 tablets for around $10)

Vitamin D

Fun fact, Vitamin D is the only vitamin your body produces due to sun exposure, sort of like a human version of photosynthesis. It's responsible for keeping your teeth, bones and muscles healthy, and yet due to the growth of indoor jobs around 50% of the world's population do not get enough sun exposure (Haq et al. 2016).

Now, most people can make up for this issue by eating vitamin D rich foods like salmon, herring, tuna, shrimp and eggs, but if you're following a vegan diet you can't eat any of these foods. With this in mind you'll have to look for some alternative sources in order to meet your recommended daily intake of 10 micrograms. Theoretically mushrooms are a great option, often containing 3-4 times the RDI per 100g serving.

However, since it's becoming more and more common for mushrooms to be grown indoors (with no exposure to sunlight) they're becoming less and less of a reliable source. I recommend either buying organic mushrooms, or checking the packaging to see if they are advertised as high in Vitamin D. Other than mushrooms, some good sources include fortified juices and milks which have about 20% RDI per cup. There are also fortified oatmeals and cereals which tend to have around 50% RDI per cup. Just like with Vitamin B-12 below, a simple bowl of fortified cereal or oats with some fortified milk can go a long way to helping you hit your RDI, and if you're really struggling you can also buy vitamin D supplement tablets for very low prices (200+ tablets for less than $10)

Iron

One of the first things you'll hear when you tell someone you're following a plant-based diet is "how do you get enough iron?" (The first thing you'll hear is "how do you get enough protein?") The reason people ask is essentially because meat is incorrectly considered to be one of your only sources of iron. The reality is that there are plenty of fantastic plant-based sources of iron, which is useful considering that it's used in the production of red blood cells, which transport oxygen around the body.

Try running a marathon without good oxygen transportation! (seriously, though, don't actually try it!) Your recommended daily intake is 8.7mg (or 14.8mg if you're on your period). Good vegan sources include beans such as kidney beans, black eyed peas and chickpeas which have 3.5-4.5mg of iron per cup. Lentils, which have 6.5mg iron per cup, and soy-based foods such as tofu, tempeh and natto, each of which provides around 6.65mg iron per cup. There's also iron in spinach, apricots and fortified cereals, so you've actually got a pretty wide selection of foods you can choose from.

Omega 3

Omega 3 is responsible for the maintenance of cell membranes, nervous system function, controlling cholesterol levels and the reduction of inflammation. If you're deficient in omega 3 you'll notice things like brittle hair and nails, as well as difficulty paying attention and difficulty sleeping, which will impact your recovery from training. This is tricky for vegans because the best sources of omega 3 tend to be oily fish.

Additionally, you also have to consider your balance of omega 3 to omega 6. Often expressed as a ratio, this balance should be somewhere in the region of 1:1 to 1:5 for optimal health, yet for most people is more like 1:20. On a plant-based diet you'll be consuming plenty of nuts and seeds, but since many of these are high in omega 6 it can push this ratio further off balance. To help top up your omega 3's and maintain a healthy omega 3 to omega 6 balance, you should make sure to include some plant-based sources of omega 3.

Great options include flax seeds, which have 2350mg of omega 3 per tablespoon, hemp seeds, which have around 2500mg per tablespoon, and chia seeds, which have around 5000mg per tablespoon. Alternatively, if you're not a huge seed fan, then walnuts could be useful as they contain 2500mg per 30g serving.

Iodine

Iodine is really important from a body composition standpoint, as it's a mineral responsible for thyroid health through the production of thyroid hormones. Too much or too little iodine can lead to metabolic issues and trouble maintaining a stable bodyweight, which can be a nightmare for predictable athletic performance. Common sources include sea fish and shellfish, but since these aren't part of a vegan diet it you'll have to look for alternatives. Some good options include various whole grains, kale, green beans, strawberries, watercress and organic potatoes, although the best options are seaweed and edible kelp, which have the highest concentrations of iodine. Putting just a small amount into a stew or soup each week can be a simple way of meeting your recommended amounts and can actually be pretty tasty! Seaweed dishes aren't common in the US and Western Europe, but are frequently used in East Asian cooking.

Essential Staple Foods and Equipment You'll Need Foods

Lentils and beans: This is a pretty broad category, but that's a good thing when it comes to keeping your diet interesting as these will be an absolute staple of your plant-based diet. They're good sources of protein as well as good sources of carbohydrates, plus they're super cheap, which is great if you're on a budget. You can buy most dried beans and lentils in big packs, which is super cost effective, but you'll have to soak them for a few hours before cooking with them. You can also buy them pre-soaked and canned, which is slightly more expensive but far more convenient. To be honest, though, at an average cost of $0.75 per can they're still an insanely cheap food source.

- black beans and kidney beans for chilli-based dishes and stir fries

- haricot and barlotti beans for stews.

- Butter beans, which make a great addition to salads.

- Green lentils are great in salads, stews and even pies.

Nuts and seeds: These are a great source of protein, carbs and healthy fats. They're also high in calories, making them a great 'on the go' snack for athletes. Just like with lentils and beans this category contains a huge range of options.

- Chia seeds and flax seeds are great sources of omega 3. You can pop them into stews, sprinkle them over salads, blend them into smoothies and bake with them.

- Cashew nuts and walnuts can be eaten on their own as high calorie snacks or used to add some real crunch and body to stir fries. They can also form well a central component in various pies and bakes.

- Macadamia nuts are rich and buttery, making them a great addition to desserts or just a tasty standalone snack.

Starches: Just like in a non-vegan kitchen, complex carbohydrates (starches) will pretty much form the cornerstone of most meals. Carbs are cheap, filling and provide the majority of your energy for athletic performance, especially when timed appropriately according to glycaemic index. A lower GI means slow digesting, slow release energy, whereas a high GI means faster digesting, faster release energy. Generally, you'll want to eat your faster digesting foods around training.

- Potatoes, both regular and sweet are great for stews, roast dinners and salads. They can also be made into delicious home fries. (Moderate to High GI)

- Wholewheat Pasta is great for tomato or vegan carbonara style dishes (Low GI)

- Brown rice has a distinct nutty taste, which makes it great alongside stir fries. (Low GI)

- White rice is great for stir fries and curry dishes. It has a moderate to Low GI making a bit better for light meals when you need to be on the move in the next hour or two. (Moderate to Low GI)

- Eggless noodles such as rice noodles can make ramen style broths packed full of flavor and nutrition. (High GI)

- Oats and breakfast cereals. Personally, I'll always have a couple of boxes of B-12, Vitamin D and Iron fortified cereals handy each week. (Low GI) Remember, though, this refers to basic oat and bran cereals, if you have a cereal with loads of added sugar, this will give it a much higher GI value.

Fruit and vegetables: No healthy diet can possibly be complete without fruit and vegetables as these are essential for providing a whole range of vitamins and minerals. Aim to eat the widest possible variety of colours, as this ensures you'll be getting a good range of phytonutrients (McManus 2019) Personally, I like to stock 3 or 4 vegetables and 2 or 3 types of fruit every week, rotating the selection every week or two for variety. So, a single week of shopping might include...

- Peppers

- Mushrooms

- Carrots

- Broccoli

- Apples

- Oranges

- Pears.

Soy-Based Products: These are great sources of protein and iron. Generally, I recommend buying the firm version, as this is the most versatile for cooking. (Silken versions are more appropriate for desserts.) Just make sure you press them first then cook them with plenty of sauce, spices or seasonings, as they can be a bit dull on their own.

- Tofu

- Tempeh

- Natto

Meat Alternatives: These can be a fantastic, quick and healthy option for your plant-based diet. Brands like Quorn and Linda McCartney are growing every year, with an expanding range of chicken, beef and fish alternatives. Personally, I think they can be a great way to ease your transition into plant-based eating. I also like that most of them can be oven cooked in 15-25 minutes, which is really handy after a long day at work. They are typically made either from soy, or from beans and vegetables, with varying amounts of protein content, so be sure to check the labels. Some examples include:

- Vege-Burgers
- Vege-Sausages
- Vege-Meatballs
- Fishless Fingers/Fishcakes
- Meatless Mince
- Seitan (hydrated gluten, really high in protein)

Authors Note: Meat-alternatives are often unfairly criticized within the vegan/plant-based community because they're processed and thus not 'natural.' To professional dieticians, this is known as the 'naturalistic fallacy.' or the mistaken idea that just because something is natural it is healthy. The reality is that dozens of all-natural products would kill you if you ate them, so something being 'natural' is no guarantee of healthiness. On the other hand, something being processed isn't necessarily bad. The water that comes from your tap has been processed to stop you getting water-borne disease like cholera, typhoid and dysentery. What I'm saying is, keep an open mind and let good quality science rather than sensationalist internet articles help you to decide which foods to include as part of your plant-based diet. If including meat based alternatives within your week of healthy eating makes adherence to a vegan diet easier, then go for it.

Dairy alternatives: Giving up dairy can be tough! Most of us are used to having milk on our cereal, eggs for breakfast and cheese on our toast. Then there's yogurts, custard, cream and even cakes that you can't have any more. With all that in mind, there's a huge range of dairy alternatives to help make this transition easier, and some of them a pretty darn tasty.

- Instead of cow's milk you can try almond milk, coconut or oat milk.

- Instead of cow's cheese you can try nut milk-based cheeses

- Instead of whipped cream from a cow you can try the version derived from coconuts

- Instead of eggs from a hen, try vegan egg alternatives made from algai, flax or chia seeds.

The options are out there, you've just got to do a little of bit of research. Personally, I've found ordering my food shopping from supermarkets online is a fantastic way to have access to the store's full range of products.

The Importance of Meal Preparation

"If you want to improve your health, build muscle or optimize your athletic performance, but don't prepare your meals, you're shooting yourself in the foot"

When it comes to eating for performance, meal preparation is going to be your best friend, and not being organized with it is going to be your worst enemy. There's nothing worse for your athletic performance, or for muscle building, than realizing you have nothing healthy and nutritious to eat and having no time to prepare anything. Yes, you can always grab a quick snack, but it's never going to support your goals in the same way that a properly balanced and prepared meal will.

All this becomes especially important when you factor real life into your sports and fitness goals. You could end up being late back from work, have extra parental responsibilities, be tired after a long and stressful day, and so and so forth. Without meal preparation you'll end up doing one of three things...

1) Ordering junk food in

2) Eating the quickest thing you can put together at home

3) Not eating at all

None of which will support your athletic goals.

3 Quick Tips for Vegan Eating on a Budget

Tip 1: Realize that a lot of vegan food is actually super cheap

There's the huge misconception that following a vegan diet is really expensive, but that isn't really correct. Let me ask you this...

"If you had to survive on a grocery budget of $5 per week, what would you buy?"

You'd probably say rice and beans, right? A kilogram bag of rice costs a $2-3, then a big pack of dried beans or half a dozen cans costs $2-3. Simple, food for a week!

Well good news, because things like rice and beans are a huge part of a vegan diet. Rice, pasta, beans, vegetables and the like are super cheap, and form the cornerstones of vegan eating. So, the next time someone tells you that following a vegan or plant-based diet is too expensive, you'll know how to correct them.

Tip 2: Compare prices for Vegan Products

If you take meat alternatives for instance, you might have a pack of 2 soy burgers costing $3, and a packet of 8 burgers costing $2.50! When it comes to vegan products, prices can range massively despite having identical contents. This can be due to brand positioning, business costs, manufacture processes and a whole other bunch of reasons. So, don't just pick up the first thing you see, take a couple of minutes to compare prices and contents. Here are a couple other examples from my experience...

•   I swapped my fortified Kellogg's raisin bran ($3 per 500g) for a store brand fortified raisin bran costing $1.75 per 750g.

•   I swapped my luxury fruit and nut mix ($3.50 for 250g) for separate bags of peanuts, walnuts, almonds and raisins, combining them together myself for a total cost of $3.79 for 600g.

Tip 3: Be flexible and use deals

The last tip I'll give you is to be flexible enough to actually benefit from instore deals and savings. Let's say that you always buy Magical Unicorn vegan butter for $3, but there's an offer on Miraculous Panda vegan butter for $1.50.

The simple pick would be the cheaper product at $1.50 (assuming both products are of equal size and tastiness) but so many people just buy the same products out of habit, even when the price differences make no sense. Personally, I used to always buy a certain vegan yogurt brand, ignoring the others, despite the fact that the brand I chose was always rising in value. Eventually I was paying three times the price of the alternative brands and decided to make a switch. Funny thing was, I ended up liking the alternative brand more, so I'd been paying over the odds for a product I liked less, just out of habit.

Chapter 10: How to Lose Fat and Build Muscle on a Plant-Based Diet

Let's talk nutritionally because that's the only way that actually matters. Sound good? Okay, we're going to not talk about your specific training regimen here. This is strictly nutrition.

Your body needs certain diet requirements to build muscle, duh. The most important is a small calorie surplus and enough protein. When you workout, you will damage your muscles, and these two factors will help your body repair your muscle tissue in a stronger way than it was before. For muscle growth, your protein intake should be between 0.8 and 1 grams/lb of body weight per day. You can absolutely get this through a vegan diet, but you're going to need to be clever. We've already gone over the reasoning behind this, so I'll keep it brief here and give you some examples you can use today.

Peanuts (26g of protein per 100g), mung beans (24g of protein per 100g), kidney beans (24g of protein per 100g), black beans (21g of protein per 100g), chickpeas (19g of protein per 100g), pumpkin seeds (19g of protein per 100g), chia seeds (17g of protein per 100g), oats (17g of protein per 100g) and lentils (9g of protein per 100g).

Eat a few servings of those through the day, and you'll get a significant amount of protein very quickly. I'd recommend also tossing in a vegan protein powder supplement, the best of which are usually pea or rice protein powder. Better yet, get one that blends both. Take one or two scoops of them per day, and you'll be fine.

Keep an eye on your calorie balance. You're going to need a slight calorie surplus to gain muscle, which might be difficult, seeing as vegan diets are not known for their ability to let someone overeat. If you're having trouble and find yourself not gaining weight consistently, consider increasing your fat intake through olive oil, which is more calorie-dense than most vegan sources of carbs or protein. If you do this, make sure you still reach your macro requirements of carbs and protein per day.

Here's the bottom line: you can build muscle and strength on a vegan diet.

Muscle Building Formula

There are a million books out there about bodybuilding because there's enough information for a million books about bodybuilding. You might have read a few of them, or you've found one of those fitness gurus or magazines that give you all sort of complex hacks and workouts that makes it mighty confusing. There's just so much information out there. I know, I've looked into it. It makes something that really isn't all that complex seem like rocket science. Here's the great news: if you're not a professional bodybuilder, you don't actually need to know everything. In fact, you need to know precisely three things, these three things that I'll tell you right now.

Train.

Eat.

Recover.

Let's go over that one more time for the people in the back. Train. Eat. Recover. Really. It's that simple. That's literally all you need to do to build muscle. I'll go a little deeper into each of these, but this is exactly as hard as it needs to be.

Train. For workouts, I'd recommend compound exercises/compound movements. Basically, instead of working for just one muscle group, you work many, including many that you just can't with other exercises. You can lift more weight—but be safe—and you'll get faster growth. The biggest of these are the barbell squat, the bench press, the military press, and the deadlift. They're best with heavyweight within reason and with fewer reps. I'll be calling these the big four because there are exactly four of them and I'm clever like that.

You're going to see an increase of strength right of the bat because your muscles will be completely surprised by these four. Great! Then, you'll plateau. Don't panic. That's exactly what is expected. It happens to everyone. When that happens, you're going to need to come up with a workout plan that enables you to get stronger when adding more weight isn't an option. Just to confirm, the very much incorrect option is to overload yourself and injure yourself. I can't even begin to emphasize how important it is to do these big four with proper form and safety.

Cardio. Personally, I hate cardio with regarding passion even though it does great stuff for you, but you need to decide what your workout goals are before doing cardio. Cardio burns calories, and if you burn too much, you won't have a that important calorie surplus, and your body just can't build muscle. If you want to pack on muscle, consider eating more or doing less cardio.

Eat. Yes, I know that people like to think of calories as awful, but you need that surplus if you're going to build muscle. Your muscles don't grow as you workout. They grow after you finish, and you need to be getting the right calories and from the right places.

Recover. The fun part for many people this is the part when your body is reeling from working out, getting the necessary fuel, and doing what you want: getting stronger and building muscle. Much of this is done when you sleep, so make sure to get seven to nine hours of uninterrupted sleep per night, at least. Less than seven, and you'll be sacrificing possible progress and maybe your health in general. It'd be pretty stupid to go through all the effort of working out, then lose it because you didn't do the easiest thing on the planet: sleep.

Bulking and Cutting

Lots of bodybuilders and athletes do this. It's two phases, bulking and cutting. Bulking is getting bigger and gaining lots of muscle and size from eating more calories, then cutting is when you try to get rid of this extra body fat by cutting calories while maintaining lean muscle mass. This actually does work, and it's a legitimate thing I would strongly consider if I was you. There's a good reason that people do this. Luckily, it's easy. Lift heavy and eat lots of calories, and you'll grow. If you don't lift heavy enough (and this varies by person), or if you don't eat enough, even if you go to the gym five times a week, this won't work.

If you're a complete beginner, your body will do both cutting and bulking at the same time because it's such a new thing. Once you get more muscle, you will have to focus more on these two actual phases. Now, I want to tell you one thing right now: don't use any meal plans from the internet. Many of them are complete garbage that will actually damage you more than helping you. Here's how you do it: calculate your TDEE, then add a certain percentage of your TDEE to get your ideal calorie count for your bulk. Then, get there by eating healthy. Don't decide that you need extra calories and go eat ice cream to get there.

What's the percentage? You'll hear both sides, with some saying to add ten percent and some saying that won't make any difference. The truth lies somewhere in the middle. If you eat way, way over your level, your body won't be able to put all those extra calories towards muscle growth, and you'll get fatter. I'd try 20%, personally. I can't tell you exactly, because this boils down to your individual metabolism. You might have to play with it a bit. If you're a skinnier person with an extremely high metabolism, you're going to need to eat more than a bigger person.

Fat Loss Formula

Right now, google fat loss diets. I'll wait. You'll find eight hundred different, super muscular, super-fit gurus telling you that all the other diets are frauds and only theirs will work, and, what's more, it'll work in no time! Yeah... right. Don't just blindly trust these people. If you want to lose weight, it's very simple. There was actually a study done where people ate literally nothing other than Twinkies and they lost weight because they ate fewer calories than they expended. Heck, if you wanted, you could lose all kinds of weight by literally just not eating, but that's not a good plan, because it's very unhealthy.

No, what you want is not to shrivel up, but to keep your healthy mass and lose fat. There's a big difference here. If you want to do it the healthy way, look at the total calorie count, sure, but look at what's actually in there. You need healthy fats, proteins, and carbs for this to work. You need to also work out during this period, or you will lose muscle along with fat.

Well, hold on, you say. I met this guy who swore he had a diet that could make him gain crazy amounts of muscle and lose all his body fat at the same time! Isn't that great? No, no, it is not because that guy is lying to you. Such a thing does not exist.

Ooh, here we go again, with another myth! The spot reduction myth. Have fat around your belly that you don't like Well, it would make sense that working on ab exercises would make belly fat go around faster than a chest exercise, right? Unfortunately, no, though that would be awesome. Some people lose fat faster than others in various places, and that's due to a little something called good genes, not the exercises they do. Another myth is that cardio will make you lose weight, which is sometimes true. If you're eating thousands of more calories than you should, you can do all the exercise you want, and you won't lose weight. You'll be putting it on.

You're going to need, for the cutting phase, a calorie deficit. You calculate this the exact same way you calculated the bulking diet, but with a difference. Obviously, you aren't going to add calories on top to lose weight. There are three classifications of calorie deficits:

- Small (10 to 15 percent below your TDEE)

- Moderate (20 to 25 percent below your TDEE)

- Large (More than 25 percent below your TDEE)

Some say that small is good. Others say that moderate is best. Very few say the large is a good plan. If you want to lose body fat fast, a moderate deficit of 20 percent below is probably your best option. If you have a faster metabolism, a smaller deficit will probably do the same thing while you sacrifice less strength while allowing you to eat more during your day. You need protein while cutting. Want to lose fat and not muscle? Protein. Normally, it's 0.8-1 gram of protein per pound of body weight.

Cheat Sheets

If you want spark an argument in your fitness and nutrition groups, bring up cheat sheets. Basically, let's say that you've been eating healthy for a week, but you really, really want to sneak in that chocolate bar at the end of the week. That's a cheat meal. It doesn't fall into your normal diet, but you really want it as a reward. Is it going to destroy you? No, of course not—as long as you keep your calories and macros in check.

I'm going to go ahead and say that 10 to 20 percent of your diet can be coming from whatever food you want, as long as it fits your total daily calories and proteins, carbs, and fats. Some people, and I've met several, can stick to a 100 percent diet. I can't. I know I can't. I would go insane. Most people would. You aren't a machine. As long as you stick to the basics of correct dieting, cheat meals are not going to cause you to get fat or lose muscle magically. Now, here's your test: you've been eating good, so you decide to eat an entire gallon of ice cream. Was that a good idea? Of course not, because you've gone way over your calorie balance.

And then, there are cheat days. Cheat days are a significantly worse idea than cheat meals because they can actually screw up the plan. If you eat five hundred calories less than your normal every day for a week, great. You can blow it all by eating badly for a day. It's just not worth it. None of us are machines, and it can be tempting to have cheat days, but you'll be shooting yourself in the foot. There are two ways to get around this problem: first, suffer. Second, make a diet that you can stick to.

Pea Protein Powder

Pea powder is made of dried yellow field pieces of fiber as a legume. It contains all the essential amino acids (except for methane). It's an excellent protein source for vegans and vegetarians. It's basically the vegan alternative to whey protein. You need protein for building muscle, and while you can get it from various foods, it's tricky and requires a good amount of planning and calculation... Or you could use pea protein powder with a balanced diet. It's completely vegan, and it's a high-quality protein and is extremely comparable to whey protein, and studies can prove it. Also, since it's not made from milk, it's an excellent choice for those who are lactose intolerant.

Don't use any kind of protein powder as your sole source of protein. Maybe get a third of your diet, a half max, of your protein from protein shakes.

Are there side effects? Nope. It's very safe. If you have preexisting kidney problems, talk to your doctor first, but studies have shown it's safe for everyone else.

How to Use Creatine?

Creatine stands out as one of the very few supplements that actually does make you see more gains. Through the magic of science, it will make you stronger, and it will cause more water retention in your muscles, which you want because it makes them appear bigger and fuller. But, who cares if it isn't safe? Luckily for us, study after study shows that it's completely safe.

But what kind? There are tons of forms, but luckily, the research is pretty obvious: creatine monohydrate is the most effective form. You'll see more expensive kinds, like creatine ethyl and Ke Alkalyn (aka, buffered creatine), but they don't have any extra benefits, and they can be more than twice the price. No, here's what you have to do— traditional creatine monohydrate supplement. Make sure you look for the Creapure trademark because they will assure you that you'll have one hundred percent pure product.

When should I take it? It doesn't matter very much, seeing as it doesn't have an instant effect. Some people like to say that you should take it after your workout. These people like to cite studies that say there is better absorption after a workout, but here's the thing: in those studies, the researchers actually declared that the difference was so tiny that it wasn't statistically relevant. You do you. You take it when you can.

Vegan Food for Energy

Theoretically, every food has calories, and calories give you energy, so it would make sense that every food would provide you with energy, with very high-calorie foods giving you the most energy. This is not quite right, unfortunately, if you consider longterm effects. Fortunately for us, there are plenty of foods that can help you get energy without compromising you in the long term. Here's what to look for!

Quality carbs. Even though they aren't vital to your survival like some other kinds of foods, they're an excellent energy source, and they're fantastic for instant energy boosts. The more intense that your workouts are, the more important carbs become. Fats provide up to 90 percent of your energy during normal activities, but when you start getting into moderate and high-intensity workouts, it shifts into overdrive and carbs start providing energy. Focus on unprocessed or minimally processed carbs like pasta, whole-grain bread, brown rice, and sweet potatoes. Bonus points for being very nutritious and being high in fiber!

Fruits. They are also carbs, but they get their own section because they hit a lot faster. If you need instant energy, you're not going to find a better source.

Coffee and tea. Well, duh. Tea takes longer to break down than coffee, so it's better for the long term, drawn-out a release of caffeine. Use them before a workout, and it'll increase your performance, but be careful—your body will get used to caffeine levels and you'll have to start drinking more and more over time.

Anything you're deficient in. If you're feeling low on energy, it could be a nutrition deficiency. I'm going to leave you with this: blood tests will tell you if you have a nutritional deficiency. If you live in cold places, you're more likely to be deficient in Vitamin D. Athletes are particularly susceptible to Vitamin C, magnesium, and iron deficiencies (which, fortunately, is an easy fix with a diet adjustment or with the right supplement). Vegan or vegetarian? You might be lacking vitamin B12 and calcium. If this is you, I have good news: these are common problems, and if you get rid of these deficiencies, you should expect a massive energy boost, and your quality of life will increase exponentially as such.

Meal Plan

Day	Breakfast	Lunch	Dinner	Snacks
1	Chocolate PB Smoothie	Cauliflower Latke	Noodles Alfredo with Herby Tofu	Beans with Sesame Hummus
2	Orange french toast	Roasted Brussels Sprouts	Lemon Couscous with Tempeh Kabobs	Candied Honey-Coconut Peanuts
3	Oatmeal Raisin Breakfast Cookie	Brussels Sprouts & Cranberries Salad	Portobello Burger with Veggie Fries	Choco Walnuts Fat Bombs
4	Berry Beetsicle Smoothie	Potato Latke	Thai Seitan Vegetable Curry	Crispy Honey Pecans (Slow Cooker)
5	Blueberry Oat Muffins	Broccoli Rabe	Tofu Cabbage Stir-Fry	Crunchy Fried Pickles
6	Quinoa Applesauce Muffins	Whipped Potatoes	Curried Tofu with Buttery Cabbage	Granola bars with Maple Syrup
7	Pumpkin pancakes	Quinoa Avocado Salad	Smoked Tempeh with Broccoli Fritters	Green Soy Beans Hummus
8	Green breakfast smoothie	Roasted Sweet Potatoes	Cheesy Potato Casserole	High Protein Avocado Guacamole
9	Blueberry Lemonade Smoothie	Cauliflower Salad	Curry Mushroom Pie	Homemade Energy Nut Bars
10	Berry Protein Smoothie	Garlic Mashed Potatoes & Turnips	Spicy Cheesy Tofu Balls	Honey Peanut Butter
11	Blueberry and chia smoothie	Green Beans with Bacon	Radish Chips	Mediterranean Marinated Olives
12	Green Kickstart Smoothie	Coconut Brussels Sprouts	Sautéed Pears	Nut Butter & Dates Granola
13	Warm Maple and Cinnamon Quinoa	Cod Stew with Rice & Sweet Potatoes	Pecan & Blueberry Crumble	Oven-baked Caramelize Plantains
14	Warm Quinoa Breakfast Bowl	Chicken & Rice	Rice Pudding	Powerful Peas & Lentils Dip
15	Banana Bread Rice Pudding	Rice Bowl with Edamame	Mango Sticky Rice	Protein "Raffaello" Candies

16	Apple and cinnamon oatmeal	Chickpea Avocado Sandwich	Noodles Alfredo with Herby Tofu	Protein-Rich Pumpkin Bowl
17	Mango Key Lime Pie Smoothie	Roasted Tomato Sandwich	Lemon Couscous with Tempeh Kabobs	Savory Red Potato-Garlic Balls
18	Spiced orange breakfast couscous	Pulled "Pork" Sandwiches	Portobello Burger with Veggie Fries	Spicy Smooth Red Lentil Dip
19	Breakfast parfaits	Cauliflower Latke	Thai Seitan Vegetable Curry	Steamed Broccoli with Sesame
20	Sweet potato and kale hash	Roasted Brussels Sprouts	Tofu Cabbage Stir-Fry	Vegan Eggplant Patties
21	Delicious Oat Meal	Brussels Sprouts & Cranberries Salad	Curried Tofu with Buttery Cabbage	Vegan Breakfast Sandwich
22	Breakfast Cherry Delight	Potato Latke	Smoked Tempeh with Broccoli Fritters	Chickpea And Mushroom Burger
23	Crazy Maple and Pear Breakfast	Broccoli Rabe	Cheesy Potato Casserole	Beans with Sesame Hummus
24	Hearty French Toast Bowls	Whipped Potatoes	Curry Mushroom Pie	Candied Honey-Coconut Peanuts
25	Chocolate PB Smoothie	Quinoa Avocado Salad	Spicy Cheesy Tofu Balls	Choco Walnuts Fat Bombs
26	Orange french toast	Roasted Sweet Potatoes	Radish Chips	Crispy Honey Pecans (Slow Cooker)
27	Oatmeal Raisin Breakfast Cookie	Cauliflower Salad	Sautéed Pears	Crunchy Fried Pickles
28	Berry Beetsicle Smoothie	Garlic Mashed Potatoes & Turnips	Pecan & Blueberry Crumble	Granola bars with Maple Syrup

Conclusion

As an athlete, it may sound like the vegan diet may not provide you the right nutrition. But I am sure after reading these recipes; you can very well debunk that myth.

Over the course of the book, I've given you a bunch of tasty and easy to cook recipes which will make sure that you get your share of protein and carbs. Remember that while being a meat free athlete isn't easy, this is hardly a reason to quit!

One of the greatest benefits of going vegan is the increased level of health you will experience and this manifests well beyond just your physique. Add to this the potent combination of healthy plant based protein and you have a winner! The vegan diet is famous for its health benefits and especially for weight loss. Many people have made a vegan diet to lose weight and have succeeded.

Lose weight, enjoy more energy, and feel good by making a difference in vegetarianism. But before starting a vegan diet, you may be looking for a healthy and healthy diet to lose weight, and there are some things you should understand.

Most people make the mistake of giving the word 'diet' a negative connotation. It is for this reason that most of them are unable to stick to a diet when they want to switch to a different lifestyle. It is important that you do not do that. Tell yourself that you are switching to a healthier lifestyle that has numerous benefits. Remember that it is okay to give yourself one cheat meal. You can consume this meal on those days when you have cravings. You should remember to never make a habit out of it. Once you begin to lead a vegan lifestyle fully, you will no longer have any meat cravings.

To be well prepared, the key is to have an unmistakable objective for the occasion, stick to individual plans and readiness procedures, remain at the time, and limit the effect of interruptions. Staying positive and hopeful, even despite misfortune, and overseeing feelings every day are extra tips that can have a major effect once rivalry shows up. For the groups who are set up for the experience, rivalries give energizing chances to exhibit capacities and are significant learning open doors for youthful athletes.

Now that you have learned the benefits of switching to a vegan lifestyle, and understand that there are ample plant-based or nut-based proteins that can help you provide your body with the necessary protein and other nutrients, it is time for you to get started with the recipes.

CPSIA information can be obtained
at www.ICGtesting.com
Printed in the USA
BVHW010355160521
607041BV00013BB/1559